theclinics.com

INFECTIOUS DISEASE CLINICS OF NORTH AMERICA

Pediatric Infectious Disease

GUEST EDITORS
Jeffrey L. Blumer, MD, PhD
Philip Toltzis, MD

CONSULTING EDITOR
Robert C. Moellering, Jr, MD

September 2005 • Volume 19 • Number 3

SAUNDERS
An Imprint of Elsevier, Inc.
PHILADELPHIA LONDON TORONTO MONTREAL SYDNEY TOKYO

W.B. SAUNDERS COMPANY
A Division of Elsevier Inc.

Elsevier, Inc., 1600 John F. Kennedy Blvd., Suite 1800, Philadelphia, PA 19103-2899.

http://www.theclinics.com

INFECTIOUS DISEASE CLINICS OF NORTH AMERICA
September 2005
Editor: Carin Davis

Volume 19, Number 3
ISSN 0891–5520
ISBN 1-4160-2669-X

Infectious Disease Clinics of North America (ISSN 0891–5520) is published in March, June, September, and December (For Post Office use only: volume 19 issue 3 of 4) by Elsevier, Inc. Corporate and editorial offices: Elsevier, Inc., 1600 John F. Kennedy Blvd., Suite 1800, Philadelphia, PA 19103-2899. Accounting and circulation offices: 6277 Sea Harbor Drive, Orlando, FL 32887-4800. Periodicals postage paid at Orlando, FL 32862, and additional mailing offices. Subscription prices are $165.00 per year for US individuals, $272.00 per year for US institutions, $83.00 per year for US students, $196.00 per year for Canadian individuals, $328.00 per year for Canadian institutions, $215.00 per year for international individuals, $328.00 per year for international institutions, and $108.00 per year for Canadian and foreign students. To receive student rate, orders must be accompanied by name of affiliated institution, date of term, and the *signature* of program/residency coordinator on institution letterhead. Orders will be billed at individual rate until proof of status is received. Foreign air speed delivery is included in all *Clinics* subscription prices. All prices are subject to change without notice. POSTMASTER: Send address changes to *Infectious Disease Clinics of North America*, W.B. Saunders Company, Periodicals Fulfillment, Orlando, FL 32887-4800. **Customer Service: 1-800-654-2452 (US). From outside of the US, call 1-407-345-4000. E-mail: hhspcs@wbsaunders.com**

Infectious Disease Clinics of North America is also published in Spanish by Editorial Inter-Médica, Junin 917, 1er A 1113, Buenos Aires, Argentina.

Reprints. For copies of 100 or more, of articles in this publication, please contact the Commercial Reprints Department, Elsevier Inc., 360 Park Avenue South, New York, New York 10010-1710. Tel. (212) 633-3813, Fax: (212) 462-1935, email: reprints@elsevier.com

Infectious Disease Clinics of North America is covered in *Index Medicus, Current Contents/Clinical Medicine, Science Citation Alert, SCISEARCH, and Research Alert.*

Printed in the United States of America.

CONSULTING EDITOR

ROBERT C. MOELLERING, Jr, MD, Herrman L. Blumgart Professor of Medical Research, Harvard Medical School; and Physician-in-Chief and Chairman, Department of Medicine, Beth Israel Deaconess Medical Center, Boston, Massachusetts

GUEST EDITORS

JEFFREY L. BLUMER, MD, PhD, Professor of Pediatrics, Case Western Reserve University School of Medicine; University Hospitals Health System, Rainbow Babies and Children's Hospital, Pediatric Pharmacology and Critical Care, Cleveland, Ohio

PHILIP TOLTZIS, MD, Associate Professor of Pediatrics, Case Western Reserve University School of Medicine; University Hospitals Health System, Rainbow Babies and Children's Hospital, Pediatric Pharmacology and Critical Care, Cleveland, Ohio

CONTRIBUTORS

DANIEL K. BENJAMIN, Jr, MD, MPH, PhD, Associate Professor, Department of Pediatrics and Duke Clinical Research Institute, Duke University Medical Center, Durham, North Carolina

SUSAN E. COFFIN, MD, MPH, Assistant Professor, Department of Pediatrics, University of Pennsylvania School of Medicine; Medical Director, Infection Prevention and Control Division of Infectious Diseases, Children's Hospital of Philadelphia, Philadelphia, Pennsylvania

PENELOPE H. DENNEHY, MD, Director, Division of Pediatric Infectious Diseases, Rhode Island Hospital; Professor, Department of Pediatrics, Brown Medical School, Providence, Rhode Island

LAURA GORI, MD, Pediatric Resident, Department of Procreative Medicine and Child Development, University of Pisa Hospital, Pisa, Italy

MICHAEL R. JACOBS, MD, PhD, Professor of Medicine, Director of Medical Microbiology, Department of Pathology, University Hospitals of Cleveland, Case Western Reserve University School of Medicine, Cleveland, Ohio

TUOMAS JARTTI, MD, Research Fellow, Department of Pediatrics, Turku University Hospital, Turku, Finland

SHELDON L. KAPLAN, MD, Professor and Vice-Chairman for Clinical Affairs, Department of Pediatrics, Baylor College of Medicine; Chief, Infectious Disease Service, Texas Children's Hospital, Houston, Texas

ETHAN G. LEONARD, MD, Assistant Professor, Department of Pediatrics, Case Western Reserve University School of Medicine; Associate Director, Residency Training Program, Division of Pediatric Infectious Diseases and Rheumatology, Rainbow Babies and Children's Hospital, Cleveland, Ohio

PIERANTONIO MACCHIA, MD, Professor of Pediatrics and Chair, Department of Procreative Medicine and Child Development, University of Pisa Hospital, Pisa, Italy

GIUSEPPE MAGGIORE, MD, Associate Professor of Pediatrics, Department of Procreative Medicine and Child Development, University of Pisa Hospital, Pisa, Italy

MIKA J. MÄKELÄ, MD, Chief, Department of Pediatrics, Skin and Allergy Hospital, Helsinki University Hospital, Helsinki, Finland

DAVID MARKENSON, MD, EMT-P, Director Pediatric Critical Care, Flushing Hospital Medical Center; Senior Investigator, National Center for Disaster Preparedness; Assistant Professor of Clinical Population and Family Health, Columbia University, Mailman School of Public Health, New York, New York

FRANCESCO MASSEI, MD, Department of Procreative Medicine and Child Development, Division of Pediatrics, University of Pisa Hospital, Pisa, Italy

GRACE A. McCOMSEY, MD, Associate Professor of Pediatrics and Medicine, Department of Pediatrics, Case Western Reserve University School of Medicine; Chief, Division of Pediatric Infectious Diseases and Rheumatology, Rainbow Babies and Children's Hospital, Cleveland, Ohio

OLLI RUUSKANEN, MD, Professor of Infectious Diseases, Department of Pediatrics, Turku University Hospital, Turku; Finland

URS B. SCHAAD, MD, Professor and Chairman, Department of Pediatrics, and Medical Director, University Children's Hospital, Basel, Switzerland

P. BRIAN SMITH, MD, Neonatal Fellow, Department of Pediatrics and Duke Clinical Research Institute, Duke University Medical Center, Durham, North Carolina

WILLIAM J. STEINBACH, MD, Assistant Professor, Department of Pediatrics, Duke University Medical Center, Durham, North Carolina

PHILIP TOLTZIS, MD, Associate Professor of Pediatrics, Case Western Reserve University School of Medicine; University Hospitals Health System, Rainbow Babies and Children's Hospital, Pediatric Pharmacology and Critical Care, Cleveland, Ohio

TIMO VANTO, MD, Consultant in Allergology, Department of Pediatrics, Turku University Hospital, Turku, Finland

JOHN V. WILLIAMS, MD, Assistant Professor, Department of Pediatrics, Division of Pediatric Infectious Diseases, Vanderbilt University Medical Center, Nashville, Tennessee

THEOKLIS E. ZAOUTIS, MD, MSCE, Assistant Professor, Department of Pediatrics, and Center for Clinical Epidemiology and Biostatistics, University of Pennsylvania School of Medicine; Director, Antimicrobial Stewardship Program, Division of Infectious Diseases, Children's Hospital of Philadelphia, Philadelphia, Pennsylvania

CONTENTS

Numerous emerging respiratory tract viruses have been identified as significant causes of acute upper and lower respiratory tract illness in children. Human metapneumovirus is a paramyxovirus discovered in 2001 in the Netherlands, with a seasonal occurrence and spectrum of clinical illness most similar to the closely related respiratory syncytial virus. Several new members of the coronavirus family have been identified, including the truly novel agent of severe acute respiratory syndrome and others that probably have been circulating undetected. Avian influenza strains have caused numerous outbreaks with high mortality, including children, and are potential causes of pandemic influenza. Several zoonotic paramyxoviruses, including Nipah and Hendra viruses, have emerged as occasional causes of severe outbreaks of respiratory tract illness in children and adults.

Diarrhea is one of the most common causes of morbidity and mortality in children worldwide. The causes of acute diarrhea in children vary with the location, time of year, and population studied. There is increasing recognition of a widening array of enteric pathogens associated with diarrheal disease. Adequate fluid and electrolyte replacement and maintenance are key to managing diarrheal illnesses. Thorough clinical and epidemiologic evaluation is needed to define the severity and type of illness, exposures, and whether the patient is immunocompromised to direct

Infection Control, Hospital Epidemiology, and Patient Safety 647
Susan E. Coffin and Theoklis E. Zaoutis

Health care–acquired infections are a major risk for hospitalized children. Similar to adult patients, children are vulnerable to infections related to medical devices. Children also are at significant risk of nosocomial transmission of common pediatric viral illnesses, such as respiratory syncytial virus and varicella. In addition, pediatric patients have unique or incompletely developed immune systems.

The Link Between Bronchiolitis and Asthma 667
Tuomas Jartti, Mika J. Mäkelä, Timo Vanto, and Olli Ruuskanen

Bronchiolitis and asthma are common wheezing illnesses of childhood. Respiratory syncytial virus is the main causative agent of bronchiolitis. Rhinovirus is the most common trigger of exacerbations of asthma, but also has been detected increasingly in young children with bronchiolitis. Reportedly, childhood asthma develops in 40% of children with a history of bronchiolitis. No convincing link has been reported between bronchiolitis and development of atopy, although atopy generally is regarded as the main risk factor for chronic asthma. This article focuses on the association between bronchiolitis and the development of asthma. The authors address the question how respiratory syncytial virus and rhinovirus infections in young children, together with genetics and immunologic immaturity, may contribute to the development of asthma.

The Expanded Spectrum of Bartonellosis in Children 691
Francesco Massei, Laura Gori, Pierantonio Macchia, and Giuseppe Maggiore

Bartonella spp cause various clinical syndromes in immunocompetent and immunocompromised hosts. Domestic cats are the natural reservoir and vectors of *B henselae*. *B henselae* infection usually occurs early in childhood, is generally asymptomatic, and in most cases revolves spontaneously. It may, however, produce a wide spectrum of clinical symptoms, the most frequent feature being cat-scratch disease. Disseminated atypical *B henselae* infection may follow cat-scratch disease after a symptom-free period or may present de novo mimicking a wide range of clinical disorders. A careful clinical history researching an intimate contact with a kitten associated with a specific serology and an abdominal ultrasound for typical hepatosplenic involvement may allow a rapid and accurate diagnosis.

Antiretroviral Therapy in HIV-Infected Children: The Metabolic Cost of Improved Survival 713
Ethan G. Leonard and Grace A. McComsey

Although highly active antiretroviral therapy (HAART) has positively altered the mortality rates in HIV-infected children, these drugs have the potential to cause significant morbidity. These drugs cause changes in fat distribution, lipid profiles, glucose homeostasis, and bone turnover. The direct relationship between duration of drug exposure and increased risk of cardiovascular disease is particularly concerning for HIV-infected infants and children, who likely will have longer cumulative exposure to HAART. It is unclear whether the metabolic effects of decades of exposure would be reversible with cessation of therapy. The benefits of HAART in HIV infection are indisputable, but the impetus to find a cure or design more tolerable therapy is clear. Infarction may replace infection as the major cause of morbidity and mortality from HIV.

The Treatment of Children Exposed to Pathogens Linked to Bioterrorism 731
David Markenson

Health care providers must understand the following regarding pathogens linked to bioterrorism: (1) the classification and qualities of possible biologic agents; (2) the natural history and management of biologic, chemical, and radiologic injuries and exposures; (3) chemical agents that may be used and their properties; (4) different types of radiologic terrorism; (5) decontamination procedures; and (6) availability of antidotes and other therapeutics.

Implications of Methicillin-Resistant *Staphylococcus aureus* as a Community-Acquired Pathogen in Pediatric Patients 747
Sheldon L. Kaplan

Methicillin-resistant *Staphylococcus aureus* is now an established community pathogen in many areas of the United States and the world. Community-acquired methicillin-resistant *S aureus* infections have changed several aspects of staphylococcal infections in children. This article discusses epidemiology, clinical manifestations, laboratory diagnosis, treatment, and prevention.

Index 759

FORTHCOMING ISSUES

December 2005

Musculoskeletal Infections
John James Ross, MD, *Guest Editor*

RECENT ISSUES

June 2005

Sexually Transmitted Infections
Jonathan M. Zenilman, MD, *Guest Editor*

March 2005

Travel and Tropical Medicine
Frank J. Bia, MD, MPH, and
David R. Hill, MD, DTM&H
Guest Editors

December 2004

Lower Respiratory Tract Infections
Thomas M. File, Jr, MD, *Guest Editor*

ELSEVIER
SAUNDERS

INFECTIOUS
DISEASE CLINICS
OF NORTH AMERICA

Infect Dis Clin N Am 19 (2005) xiii–xv

Preface

Pediatric Infectious Disease

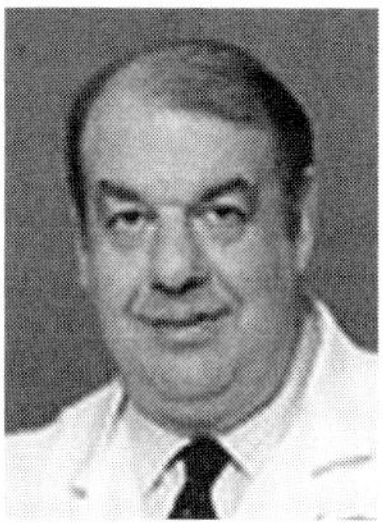

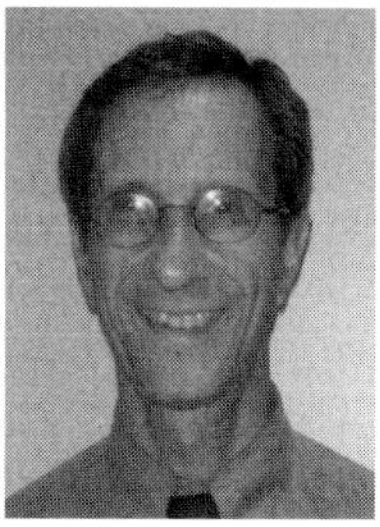

Jeffrey L. Blumer, MD, PhD   Philip Toltzis, MD
Guest Editors

This issue of the *Infectious Disease Clinics of North America* includes topics that are of current interest and importance in pediatric infectious diseases. We are delighted to have engaged a group of authors who are accomplished and widely published in each of their topics. It has long been recognized that from the medical standpoint, children are not simply small adults. Many diseases are specific to this age group, and illnesses that occur in both children and adults frequently have manifestations that are unique when they occur in the young. This is especially true for infectious diseases.

The topics discussed in this issue can be roughly categorized into three groups. The first describes the clinical appearance of emerging pediatric infections. Among these is Williams' article on newly defined viral respiratory tract pathogens in infants and children. Most prominent among these is metapneumovirus, although severe acute respiratory syndrome and the Netherlands coronaviruses and avian influenza virus in children also are described. Dennehy extensively reviews viral, bacterial, and parasitic causes of pediatric diarrheal syndromes, which together prompt an enormous number of sick child visits in industrialized nations and which remain among the most frequent causes of mortality in infants in the developing world. Massei and colleagues collate the many protean manifestations of Bartonellosis in children, from typical cat-scratch disease to the more

0891-5520/05/$ - see front matter
doi:10.1016/j.idc.2005.06.002

unusual syndromes that are beginning to emerge now that the accurate diagnosis of this infection is widely available. Kaplan presents recent data on the explosive occurrence of community-acquired methicillin-resistant *Staphylococcus aureus* in children and on the increasing breadth and severity of this infection in pediatrics, drawing on his extensive personal experience in Houston and data culled from other areas of the country.

Other articles concentrate on issues surrounding antimicrobial use in children. The incidence of fungal infections in very low birth weight newborns continues to increase as modern neonatal intensive care allows the survival of infants of younger and younger gestational age. Benjamin and colleagues offer the most current data on the use of the amphotericin preparations and the newer azoles and echinocandins in this population. Schaad discusses the use of quinolones in pediatrics, offering a reasoned analysis of the strength of the data suggesting a connection between their use and the incidence of arthropathy in young children, and describing their application in selected pediatric populations. As in adult HIV infection, highly active anti-retroviral therapy has transformed pediatric HIV infection into a chronic disease in which the side effects of the therapies often supercede the symptoms from the disease; Leonard and McComsey review the small but growing body of data examining the effects of long-term use of anti-HIV drugs in children. Finally, Markenson reviews the treatment of agents of bioterrorism in children, highlighting the aspects of these treatment schedules that differ from those applied to adults.

A third group of articles discusses epidemiologic issues pertinent to pediatric infectious diseases. Few recent events in pediatrics have been as important as the introduction of the conjugate pneumococcal vaccines in the routine pediatric immunization schedule, but has it made a difference? The review by Toltzis and Jacobs describes how this vaccine has changed the epidemiology of invasive and noninvasive pneumococcal infection in young children and their adult contacts. Asthma remains one of the most prevalent causes of morbidity in pediatrics; the link between infectious bronchiolitis in infancy and the incidence of reactive airway disease in later childhood has been debated for over a decade. The article by Ruuskanen and colleagues discusses the underlying pathophysiology that makes this association credible and catalogs and critiques the many studies purporting to show this connection. Coffin and Zaoutis offer a primer on infection control in a pediatric hospital, emphasizing the differences between the epidemiology and containment of nosocomial infections in children and adults.

These articles reflect many of the most topical issues that have appeared in pediatric infectious diseases over the past several years. They frequently draw together information that heretofore has not been presented or critiqued in a single publication. Together they should provide the reader with current information to confront some of the most important issues emerging in pediatric infections diseases today.

Jeffrey L. Blumer, MD, PhD
Philip Toltzis, MD
University Hospitals Health System
Rainbow Babies and Children's Hospital
Pediatric Pharmacology and Critical Care
11100 Euclid Avenue
Cleveland, OH 44106-6010, USA

E-mail addresses: jeffrey.blumer@uhhs.com (J.L. Blumer),
pxt2@case.edu (P. Toltzis)

ELSEVIER
SAUNDERS

Infect Dis Clin N Am 19 (2005) 569–584

INFECTIOUS DISEASE CLINICS OF NORTH AMERICA

The Clinical Presentation and Outcomes of Children Infected with Newly Identified Respiratory Tract Viruses

John V. Williams, MD

Assistant Professor, Department of Pediatrics, Division of Pediatric Infectious Diseases, Vanderbilt University Medical Center, D-7235 Medical Center North, 1161 21st Avenue South, Nashville, TN, 37232-2581, USA

Lower respiratory infection (LRI) is a leading cause of morbidity and mortality in children worldwide [1]. Upper respiratory infection (URI) is associated with significant societal costs for children in terms of lost school days and accounts for numerous health care visits, including unnecessary antibiotic prescriptions. Viral URI also commonly is associated with acute otitis media (AOM) in children, which is the most frequent diagnosis leading to antibiotic prescriptions for young children. Classic epidemiologic studies using culture and serologic methods have determined many of the etiologic agents of these common infections, such as respiratory syncytial virus (RSV), parainfluenza viruses (PIV), influenza virus, coronaviruses, and rhinoviruses [2,3]. These studies have been unable to identify a specific virus, however, in greater than 50% of such infections using traditional methods of viral culture, serology, and newer rapid antigen assays. In recent years, several novel respiratory viruses associated with acute respiratory tract illness (ARI) in humans have been identified. Some of these viruses, including human metapneumovirus (hMPV), human coronavirus–Netherlands (HCoV-NL), and human coronavirus–Hong Kong (HCoV-HK), likely have been circulating undetected for decades at least and are better described as emerging, rather than entirely new. Other viruses, including the severe acute respiratory syndrome–coronavirus (SARS-CoV), avian-derived influenza A strains, and Hendra and Nipah viruses, seem to be of more recent zoonotic origin, however, and truly are new pathogens. The distinction has important public health implications because of the effects of preexisting immunity in the populace as a whole.

E-mail address: john.williams@vanderbilt.edu

doi:10.1016/j.idc.2005.05.009

id.theclinics.com

Human metapneumovirus

Discovery

Researchers in the Netherlands reported the finding of a novel paramyxovirus associated with respiratory tract disease in 2001 [4]. The Dutch group collected numerous unidentified virus isolates, mostly from children, over a 20-year period that grew poorly in cell culture. Electron micrograph and biochemical studies of the virus showed that it was pleomorphic with a lipid envelope, consistent with a paramyxovirus. Elegant reverse transcription polymerase chain reaction (RT-PCR) experiments yielded a genomic sequence from the virus that identified it as a member of the Paramyxoviridae family, which contains many classic childhood viruses, including mumps, measles, PIV, and RSV. The gene order of the new virus was related most closely to avian pneumovirus, the sole previous member of the metapneumovirus genus. Avian pneumovirus was discovered in 1979 and is an important agricultural pathogen, causing major economic losses owing to severe respiratory disease in commercial poultry flocks. The new human metapneumovirus was unable to infect chickens and turkeys, however, and this combined with sequence comparison showed that it was a distinct human pathogen. The Dutch group also conducted serologic testing on archived human serum samples from the 1950s and found that 100% of subjects older than age 5 years were seropositive for hMPV, suggesting a high rate of infection early in life and showing that hMPV had been circulating for at least 50 years.

Diversity

hMPV has a negative-sense, single-stranded RNA genome similar to other paramyxoviruses, with a lipid envelope containing membrane proteins. Partial gene sequences for many hMPV strains worldwide are now available, and phylogenetic analysis of these sequences define two major genetic subgroups of hMPV, A and B, each with two minor subgroups. These are described presently as genogroups; it has not been shown in humans that they are antigenically distinct. In one large prospective study, primary infection during infancy was associated with LRI and subsequent infections with URI, showing that reinfection with hMPV occurs [5]. It is unclear whether this is due to infections with different subgroups that do not induce cross-protective immunity or, more likely, as is the case with RSV, to partial immunity induced by primary infection that protects the lower but not the upper respiratory tract against subsequent infection. There are no data in humans to show that infection with a virus from one subgroup protects against reinfection with a virus from a different subgroup. Animal studies suggest, however, that there is cross-protective immunity in hamsters and primates between hMPV subgroups that protects the lungs against reinfection [6,7]. These studies have important implications for the development of candidate vaccines and prophylactic antibodies against hMPV similar to palivizumab, a monoclonal antibody licensed for immunoprophylaxis against RSV for premature infants at high risk for severe disease.

Epidemiology of human metapneumovirus in children

Initial epidemiologic studies of hMPV were primarily retrospective RT-PCR analyses of diagnostic virology laboratory specimens that were previously negative for other viruses [8–10]. The percentage of hMPV detection varied from 6% to 15%, with hospitalization most prominent in infants and elderly patients. A prospective study of 587 Hong Kong children (≤18 years old) hospitalized for LRI over a 13-month period detected hMPV in 6% of the children compared with 8% for RSV and 8% for influenza virus [11]. Canadian investigators detected hMPV in 12 of 208 (6%) children younger than 3 years old hospitalized for ARI [12]. A prospective study of more than 2000 previously healthy outpatient infants and children in Tennessee found that 12% of all LRI in that cohort was attributable to hMPV [5]. In that 25-year longitudinal study, there was substantial variation in the annual prevalence of hMPV, ranging from none to 31% of otherwise negative samples in a given year. hMPV is rarely detected in nasal washes from asymptomatic patients [5,10].

Studies conducted over multiple seasons show that the annual prevalence of hMPV varies from year to year, suggesting periodic epidemics, and that strains from different subgroups frequently circulate simultaneously in the same season. In temperate zones, the seasonal peak of hMPV infections occurs in late winter and spring months, slightly later than the peak of RSV infections but overlapping substantially with the RSV season.

Studies of children hospitalized for ARI in diverse regions have found rates of hMPV associated with 6% to 40% of ARI in a given season [12–27]. The average prevalence in most pediatric populations with ARI studied is approximately 5% to 10% overall, although it may be much higher during the peak months of hMPV circulation. With few exceptions, hMPV ranks after RSV in most studies and has prevalence comparable to that of influenza virus and PIV.

Hospitalization of children for hMPV infection occurs primarily in the first year of life, although many studies reported that the peak age of hospitalization for hMPV is 6 to 12 months of age [10–12,14–16,21–26], significantly later than the 2-month peak age of hospitalization for RSV. Whether this age range reflects a difference in the decline of maternal antibodies, later acquisition of hMPV infection, or developmental airway physiology is not known. Boys are at greater risk for LRI with hMPV infection than girls, similar to RSV.

hMPV may be more severe in patients with underlying medical conditions. Many hMPV studies are of hospitalized patients and subject to selection bias. Nonetheless, 30% to 85% of children hospitalized with hMPV have chronic conditions, such as asthma, chronic lung disease secondary to prematurity, congenital heart disease, or cancer. Although most studies were not prospective, the rate of chronic disease was generally higher in hMPV-infected children than in RSV-infected children [10, 12,16,17,22–25]. A multicenter prospective study examined 641 children younger than 5 years old hospitalized for ARI or fever and found that 54% of children hospitalized with hMPV had underlying conditions versus 29% of RSV-infected patients ($P < .05$) [25].

Clinical presentation

hMPV is associated with a variety of respiratory symptoms and diagnoses. Children with hMPV infection typically present with URI symptoms, such as rhinorrhea, cough, and fever. The duration of symptoms before seeking medical attention is usually less than 1 week, and limited data suggest that children may shed virus for 1 to 2 weeks [5,10,19]. Symptoms such as conjunctivitis, vomiting, diarrhea, and rash are reported occasionally, but are not prominent in most studies. Only one study detected hMPV by RT-PCR in patients' serum [14], suggesting that similar to RSV, hMPV infection is limited to the respiratory tract. The clinical LRI syndromes associated with hMPV are bronchiolitis, croup, pneumonia, and asthma exacerbation. In the Tennessee study of previously healthy outpatients, the hMPV-infected children were diagnosed with bronchiolitis (59%), croup (18%), asthma (14%), and pneumonia (8%) [5]. In that prospective study, however, hMPV was less likely to be associated with croup than PIV and less likely to be associated with pneumonia than influenza virus. A similar spectrum of diagnoses is seen in most studies of hMPV-associated LRI, and signs and symptoms of hMPV infection overlap sufficiently with the signs and symptoms of other common respiratory viruses that reliable distinction cannot be made clinically.

In a study of more than 2400 distinct episodes of URI in previously healthy outpatient children, hMPV was associated with URI at rates similar to RSV, PIV, and influenza virus (John V. Williams, MD, et al, unpublished data). Of the children, 54% also were diagnosed with AOM, suggesting that hMPV is associated with a substantial proportion of AOM in otherwise healthy children. AOM is the most common reason for antibiotic prescription to children, and URI and AOM have significant economic impacts owing to time lost from school and work. hMPV likely has substantial medical and economic effects nationally. The only published study to examine the socioeconomic impact of hMPV directly was an Italian study of 42 hMPV-infected children seen in the emergency department in which questionnaires were administered to subjects' parents [26]. In 12% of subjects' households, other family members had similar illnesses. Parents reported a median of 4 lost working days (range 2–10), and older children reported median 4 lost school days (range 3–15). These findings were similar for children infected with RSV or influenza virus in the same study population.

Human metapneumovirus in high-risk pediatric populations

Several investigators have examined a potential relationship between hMPV infection and asthma. A prospective Australian study of outpatient children with asthma did not find an association between hMPV and asthma exacerbations [28], whereas a large prospective study of 2000 outpatient children found a highly significant association between hMPV and the diagnosis of acute asthma exacerbation [5]. A Finnish study found elevated interleukin-8 in nasal secretions from hMPV-infected infants [29], whereas another study from Argentina found decreased interleukin-8 and other cytokines in nasal washes of hMPV-infected infants compared with infants infected with RSV [30]. All such studies are complicated by the difficulty of assigning the diagnosis of asthma during infancy, when acute wheezing associated with viral infections is common.

hMPV is capable of causing severe and even fatal infections in immunocompromised hosts. There are two reports of fatal infection attributed to hMPV in cancer patients, a 33-year-old woman with leukemia who was 7 days status post hematopoietic stem cell transplant and a 17-month-old girl with relapsed leukemia [31,32]. The 17-month-old patient had had another unexplained LRI 1 year previously during chemotherapy for leukemia. Postmortem RT-PCR on respiratory samples from both illnesses detected hMPV in both, but from two distinct strains. Studies the author's group is conducting in adult and pediatric patients with cancer, including hematopoietic stem cell transplant recipients, suggest that hMPV is a relatively common cause of acute respiratory infection in these patients, with significant morbidity and mortality (John V. Williams, MD, et al, unpublished data). Further long-term prospective studies are needed to characterize fully the extent and severity of disease secondary to hMPV in immunocompromised children.

Coinfections with human metapneumovirus and other viruses

All epidemiologic studies of hMPV that have tested for other viruses have found coinfection rates of 5% to 17%, usually with RSV, and most have not noted more severe disease in these coinfected patients. A few studies of hospitalized patients have noted much higher coinfection rates of 30% to 60% [15,29,33–35], some of these authors suggesting that hMPV infections may be more severe if another virus is present. One British group addressed this question by using a nested RT-PCR assay to test bronchoalveolar lavage fluid from 30 intubated infants with RSV infection and detected hMPV in 21 of 30 (70%) [36]. The authors subsequently used the same nested assay to test respiratory specimens from children admitted to the pediatric intensive care unit (ICU) and the general wards. hMPV and RSV coinfection was detected in 18 of 25 (72%) pediatric ICU patients and 15 of 171 (9%) general ward patients [37]. The authors concluded that dual infection with RSV and hMPV was associated with severe bronchiolitis. A Connecticut study of 46 inpatients with either mild or severe RSV disease found no coinfections with hMPV, however [38]. Whether these conflicting findings are due to methodologic differences or geographic variability in circulating virus strains is unknown. Further prospective studies are needed to clarify the nature of disease associated with coinfections.

Coronaviruses

Human coronaviruses were discovered in the 1960s by researchers studying the etiology of URI in children and young adults [39]. Three major serologic groups of coronaviruses have been described. Two prototypic human viruses, each belonging to a different serologic group, originally were detected in patients who presented with URI. The group I strain, 229E, and group II strain, OC43, were the only extensively studied human coronaviruses until the identification of SARS-CoV in 2003. Coronaviruses are difficult to cultivate in tissue cell culture, so most epidemiologic studies have been based on serologic methods and likely have underestimated the extent of disease associated with human coronavirus. Early, large epidemiologic studies in the United States noted that human coronaviruses 229E and OC43 caused numerous respiratory infections with an incidence that peaked in late winter or early spring. In addition, the predominant type of coronavirus infection changed every 2 to 3 years, with the two identified human coronaviruses causing about 15% of URI, but ranging from 1% to 35% depending on the specific year [39]. The human coronaviruses originally were thought to cause only URI until the discovery of patients with pneumonia during outbreaks of human coronavirus [40]. Numerous studies now have described the role of human coronaviruses OC43 and 229E in LRI in young children [41–47].

Severe acute respiratory syndrome–coronavirus

In fall 2002, a mysterious new respiratory illness appeared in the Guangdong province of China. The illness was associated with hypoxia and rapid respiratory failure and was designated as SARS, although there were other systemic manifestations of disease. Although a subset of SARS cases also had hMPV and other viruses detected, a novel coronavirus (SARS-CoV) was determined to be the primary etiology of SARS [48–50]. Between November 2002 and July 2003, the SARS-CoV infected more than 8000 people and caused almost 800 deaths in 32 countries. Serologic evidence of previous infection in healthy humans was not detected, suggesting that SARS-CoV had emerged recently in the human population. A coronavirus with more than 99% nucleotide homology to SARS-CoV was isolated from Himalayan palm civets and raccoon dogs found in live animal markets in Guangdong, suggesting these as possible animal reservoirs [51].

The primary manifestation of SARS-CoV infection in adults is febrile LRI, with diffuse lung involvement and profound hypoxia. Other organs are affected, however, and diarrhea, lymphopenia, and hepatic abnormalities have been described. Overall mortality in adults is 10% to 17% [52]. The disease seems to have a much milder course and more favorable outcome in children, however. The first reported series of 10 children with SARS noted no deaths [53]. All children had fever and lymphopenia, and 9 of 10 had abnormal chest radiographs. All received corticosteroids and defervesced within 48 hours. Only 1 older child required mechanical ventilation.

Another institution in Hong Kong reported on 21 patients with a mean age of 11 years (range 10 months–17 years) [54]. All of the children presented with fever, and most had cough. Younger children were more likely to present with rhinorrhea and cough, whereas children older than 12 years were more likely to complain of malaise, myalgias, chills, and rigors. Although 57% of children had lymphopenia at presentation, 90% of children developed lymphopenia during the illness. Older children had generally more severe disease compared with younger children. Children older than 12 years were more likely to have higher fever for longer duration, develop thrombocytopenia, require steroid therapy, and have chest radiograph progression. Many children in both age groups had mild chemical hepatitis that resolved. All children developed radiographic abnormalities during the course of the illness, most commonly unilateral focal opacity, with occasional multifocal or bilateral opacities. Of the children, 86% had progression of the radiographic findings during the illness, but all had resolved by 2 weeks. Only 2 patients required supplemental oxygen, and none required mechanical ventilation.

A subsequent study reported 44 children with serologically confirmed SARS, including many from the two previous reports [55]. Half were male; the mean age was 12 years (range 50 days–18 years). All children presented with fever, and 64% presented with cough. Nausea and vomiting also were common. Younger children were more likely to have rhinorrhea, whereas older children were more likely to experience malaise, headache, and myalgia. None of the children had wheezing on physical examination, and few had crepitations. Three quarters of the children had lymphopenia at presentation, and 86% developed lymphopenia during their illness. Other hematologic abnormalities present during the course of infection included neutrophilia in 52%, thrombocytopenia in 27%, and anemia in 5%. Half of all patients had transient elevations of alanine aminotransferase and lactate dehydrogenase, and 39% had prolonged activated partial thromboplastin time, although none of the children had clinical jaundice or bleeding. Nine patients developed hypoxia; five of these were cared for in the ICU, and three were mechanically ventilated. Forty-two children were treated with ribavirin, and 37 were treated with steroids. Although there was no control group, a close temporal association was observed between steroid administration and clinical and radiologic improvement. None of the children died. There were 10 deaths among the adult family members of this pediatric cohort, emphasizing the difference in mortality between children and adults.

One study examined 47 serologically confirmed pediatric SARS cases 6 months after their acute illness [56]. Mild residual changes were seen on high-resolution chest CT in 34%. Younger children who had not required oxygen during acute illness were more likely to have normal studies. Four children had mild residual abnormalities measured by pulmonary function testing, but none of the children had residual clinical symptoms.

Maternal-fetal transmission of SARS-CoV has not been documented, although only one study addressed this important pediatric issue [57]. Five infants born to mothers with SARS were tested extensively by RT-PCR and viral culture on multiple body fluids, routine laboratory tests and chest radiographs, and serologic testing. No evidence for SARS-CoV infection was found in any of the infants. Two infants had gastrointestinal complications that may have been related to prematurity.

SARS-CoV infections in children seem to be relatively mild compared with adults. Two patterns of illness are seen. Younger children present with more prominent rhinorrhea, cough, and often diarrhea, whereas older children present with malaise, myalgias, chills, and rigors similar to adult disease. Fever, lymphopenia, and radiographic abnormalities are prominent at all ages. In contrast to other common respiratory viruses, male sex did not seem to be a risk factor for more severe disease because boys and girls were equally represented among hospitalized patients. Although older children are more likely to have hypoxia and a prolonged course, virtually all children recover completely without significant long-term sequelae.

Human coronavirus–Netherlands

Since the discovery of SARS-CoV, two groups in the Netherlands almost simultaneously published the discovery of another human coronavirus tentatively named *HCoV-NL*. HCoV-NL originally was cultured from respiratory specimens collected from infants with bronchiolitis [58]. Subsequently, Van der Hoek et al [58] tested respiratory specimens of hospitalized patients and outpatients collected from December 2002 to August 2003 and detected seven HCoV-NL-positive specimens in patients with ARI. Overall, 7 of 614 samples (1%) tested positive, but 7% of samples collected during January contained HCoV-NL RNA. Five of the seven samples were from infants, with a mean age of 8 months (range 4–11 months), three with URI and two with LRI. HCoV-NL was detected in specimens only from December through February. Sequencing of the isolates showed that HCoV-NL is a group I coronavirus most closely related to 229E. Another group in the Netherlands, which had discovered the virus independently, detected HCoV-NL in 4 of 139 (3%) respiratory samples [59]. The patients were three infants age 3 to 4 months and a 10-year-old child. All had presented with rhinorrhea, fever, and cough, and three had underlying conditions.

Canadian researchers tested specimens previously negative for other viruses collected from patients with ARI from several provinces and detected HCoV-NL in 19 of 525 (4%) [60]. Of these, 8 were in children younger than 5 years old, in whom the rate was higher (8 of 110, 7%). HCoV-NL was detected from January through March, but in only 1 of 2 study years. This is similar to OC43 and 229E, which are known to cause epidemics in 2- to 3-year cycles. The HCoV-NL-infected children were 85% male and presented with URI and LRI illnesses, including bronchiolitis.

Investigators in the United States screened 1265 specimens from children younger than 5 years old collected over 1 year, who previously had been negative for other viruses, and detected HCoV-NL by RT-PCR in 79 of 1265 (6%) [61]. Nine of 76 (12%) were coinfected with another virus, most with RSV. HCoV-NL was detected predominantly in the months of January and February; 67 patients had HCoV-NL detected as a sole agent. Eleven of these patients had been hospitalized since birth in the neonatal ICU and potentially had nosocomial infections. The mean age of the HCoV-NL-infected children was 6.5 months (range 1 day–5 years). Sixty-three percent were younger than 1 year old, 34% were younger than 3 months old, and 62% were male. The most common presenting signs and symptoms in non–neonatal ICU patients were cough in 77%, rhinorrhea in 68%, fever and tachypnea in 54%, and adventitious lung findings in 43%. One third of these children had hypoxia, wheezing, or retractions. Twenty of 31 had abnormal chest radiographs, mostly with peribronchial cuffing. Information on clinical diagnoses, duration of hospitalization, treatment, and outcome was not provided. The clinical description of these children, winter occurrence, and chest radiograph findings suggest, however, an illness consistent with typical viral bronchiolitis caused by RSV or hMPV. Further prospective studies are needed to clarify the clinical presentation and course of illness with HCoV-NL. A major limitation of all of these studies is that no control groups were included to examine asymptomatic carriage and strengthen the case for a causal relationship between HCoV-NL and ARI.

Avian influenza virus

Influenza has been well described as an important respiratory pathogen in young children, with the greatest morbidity and rates of hospitalization in young infants [62,63]. The major hemagglutinin types associated with disease in humans are H1 and H3, and these are the most important protective antigens. Severe pandemics of influenza occur as a result of major antigenic changes in the hemagglutinin (antigenic shift) caused by reassortment of one or more of the genomic segments, introducing novel strains into circulation. The lack of preexisting immunity in most or all of the population allows pandemics to occur, and disease may be more severe because of the lack of even partially protective immunity. Avian influenza viruses carry novel hemagglutinins, such as H5, H7, and H9, but generally do not replicate efficiently in humans. Reassortment with human strains can allow a recombinant virus to emerge, however, that is highly pathogenic and infectious for human hosts. This reassortment between human and avian strains is though to occur primarily in pigs, which are susceptible to infection by both strains. Numerous outbreaks of such novel avian influenza viruses have been reported in recent years. Almost all have been linked epidemiologically to close contact with poultry, chiefly chickens or ducks, and human-to-human transmission has been documented rarely.

Mild respiratory disease in two children caused by reassortment human-avian influenza strains was reported in the Netherlands in 1994 [64]. In 1997, a 3-year-old boy in Hong Kong died as a result of acute respiratory failure and multiorgan system dysfunction secondary to an H5 influenza strain. Genetic analysis of the virus showed that it was an avian strain [65]. In that outbreak, five other children younger than age 18 were infected. A 13-year-old girl died of acute respiratory failure and multiorgan system dysfunction, a 2-year-old boy was hospitalized for 3 days with pneumonia, and three other children experienced uneventful URI. Twelve cases were reported, with more severe disease and a higher fatality rate in the adults [66].

Several sporadic outbreaks of avian influenza have occurred since the 1997 cases. There were two confirmed H5N1 cases and one probable H5N1 case in Hong Kong in February 2003 [67]. A 33-year-old man developed fatal progressive respiratory failure, and his 8-year-old son recovered from respiratory disease after a prolonged hospitalization. Both patients had profound lymphopenia, hypoxia, and consolidation of chest radiographs. The family had a 7-year-old daughter who had died of a febrile pneumonia 1 week before the father's illness, but she had not been tested for influenza. Two cases of H9N2 avian influenza infection of humans occurred in Hong Kong, one a child, with typical influenza symptoms of fever, rhinorrhea, and cough [68]. Both patients fully recovered. From January to March 2003, there were 34 cases of confirmed H5N1 infection in humans in Thailand and Vietnam [69,70]. Of the five laboratory-confirmed cases in Thailand with clinical data provided, four were boys age 6 to 7 years. All had fever, cough, and tachypnea. Lymphopenia and elevated transaminases were common. All patients had abnormalities on chest radiograph consisting of focal consolidation or multifocal opacities, and all required mechanical ventilation. These 4 children all died, and overall mortality in the Thailand outbreak was 8 of 12 (67%). In January 2004, 10 H5N1 cases were reported in Vietnam. Eight patients were 18 years old or younger, with a mean age of 12, and the youngest child was 5. All patients had fever, tachypnea, cough, and hypoxia. Five had diarrhea, and none of the children had myalgia, rash, or conjunctivitis. Prominent laboratory abnormalities included lymphopenia, thrombocytopenia, and elevated transaminases. All had focal consolidation or extensive infiltrates on chest radiographs, which worsened significantly during the course of illness. All developed respiratory failure requiring mechanical ventilation, and seven of eight children died, despite aggressive supportive care and treatment with oseltamivir, ribavirin, or steroids for acute respiratory distress syndrome.

Subsequently, two other children were identified with probable or confirmed H5N1 infection during the same outbreak [71]. A 9-year-old girl presented with fever, watery diarrhea, hypotension, and depressed level of consciousness. Laboratory studies, including cerebrospinal fluid, were normal. She had rapidly progressive hemodynamic instability and coma and died the next day. Eight days later, her 4-year-old brother developed fever, headache, vomiting, and severe watery diarrhea. His initial diagnostic studies were remarkable only for elevated transaminases. He developed pneumonia and depressed mental status, became comatose, and died of respiratory failure 5 days after admission. During the course of his illness, he developed lymphopenia, thrombocytopenia, and bilateral infiltrates on chest radiograph. Cerebrospinal fluid was remarkable only for elevated protein. He was given the diagnosis of encephalitis, and postmortem testing detected H5N1 influenza by RT-PCR in cerebrospinal fluid, serum, and throat and rectal swabs, and culture of cerebrospinal fluid grew H5N1 influenza virus. No testing was done on his sister, but it is highly likely that she also was infected with H5N1. Neither child presented with respiratory symptoms, and the sister never had respiratory disease. Both had had significant exposure to ducks and chickens.

Avian influenza virus strains have the potential to be highly pathogenic in humans, and disease seems to be at best only slightly less severe in children. Most cases, but not all, have clear exposure to domestic fowl. Human-to-human transmission is rare. Most children present with fever, rhinorrhea, and cough, and lymphopenia, thrombocytopenia, and elevated transaminases are common. Some children can present with gastrointestinal disease alone. There are insufficient data to determine the efficacy of the neuraminidase inhibitors, oseltamivir and zanamivir, or the adamantanes, amantadine and rimantidine. The potential for widespread pandemics exists, and it is likely that more cases will be seen in sporadic outbreaks.

Hendra and Nipah viruses

Novel paramyxoviruses have been identified in Australia and Malaysia associated with acute febrile encephalitis and respiratory tract disease in humans. Hendra virus infected three adults, two of whom died with pneumonitis and multiorgan failure, and numerous horses [72]. No pediatric cases have been reported yet. The closely related Nipah virus was identified during an outbreak in Malaysia during 1998–1999 that included more than 250 patients [73]. Most presented with fever, headache, and vomiting, and half had a depressed level of consciousness; 14% of the patients had cough, but respiratory or multiorgan system disease was less prominent than neurologic disease. A variety of neurologic symptoms were noted, primarily related to brainstem and spinal cord involvement. One third of the patients died, and 28% of the survivors had neurologic sequelae. Most of the patients were men who were pig farmers, and only a few children were affected, the youngest age 13 years. In Bangladesh in 2001 and 2003, there were outbreaks of a Nipah-like virus involving 13 and 12 patients [74]. Several children, the youngest age 4 years, were infected in each outbreak, and the overall mortality was 67%. Similar to the Malaysian outbreak, the most prominent symptoms were fever, headache, vomiting, and an altered level of consciousness. Respiratory illness was much more common in the Bangladesh cases, however, with 64% having cough and dyspnea. Whether the increased involvement of the respiratory tract was due to differences between virus strains is not known. Epidemiologic investigations identified fruit bats of the *Pteropus* genus as asymptomatic carriers of Hendra and Nipah viruses and possible animal reservoirs. Further outbreaks have not been reported, and these viruses have not yet been detected in other geographic regions. Their apparent virulence for humans warrants further research and surveillance for similar viruses in other populations.

Summary

Several emerging or truly novel respiratory tract viruses affecting children have been described in recent years. The most important of these novel viruses in children seems to be hMPV. hMPV is a common cause of URI and LRI in healthy infants and children and those with underlying medical conditions. Clinical disease resulting from hMPV is most similar to that caused by RSV. hMPV may be more severe in children with underlying conditions and has been associated with fatal disease in immunocompromised hosts. Further outbreaks of SARS-CoV have not occurred, but children younger than 12 years old with SARS have a relatively mild course and good prognosis. Older children are more likely to present with severe respiratory disease similar to adults. The coronavirus HCoV-NL seems to be a less common cause of ARI, but its full epidemiology and clinical spectrum of disease have not been defined. The emergence of avian influenza viruses in humans is highly concerning for potential pandemics. Avian influenza viruses have extreme virulence in children, with multiorgan disease and high mortality. Suspicion for the presence of avian influenza relies heavily on epidemiologic risk factors, such as exposure to poultry or travel to endemic regions. Nipah and Hendra viruses have been associated with severe encephalitis and pneumonitis in children and adults, although these viruses have not yet been detected in Europe or the Americas.

References

[1] World Health Organization. Acute respiratory infection in children. Available at: http://www.who.int/fch/depts/cah/resp_infections/en/. Accessed January 10, 2005.

[2] Glezen WP, Loda FA, Clyde WA Jr, et al. Epidemiologic patterns of acute lower respiratory disease of children in a pediatric group practice. J Pediatr 1971;78:397–406.

[3] Henderson FW, Clyde WA Jr, Collier AM, et al. The etiologic and epidemiologic spectrum of bronchiolitis in pediatric practice. J Pediatr 1979;95:183–90.

[4] van den Hoogen BG, DeJong JC, Groen J, et al. A newly discovered human pneumovirus isolated from young children with respiratory tract disease. Nat Med 2001;7:719–24.

[5] Williams JV, Harris PA, Tollefson SJ, et al. Human metapneumovirus and lower respiratory tract disease in otherwise healthy infants and children. N Engl J Med 2004;350:443–50.

[6] MacPhail M, Schickli JH, Tang RS, et al. Identification of small-animal and primate models for evaluation of vaccine candidates for human metapneumovirus (hMPV) and implications for hMPV vaccine design. J Gen Virol 2004;85:1655–63.

[7] Skiadopoulos MH, Biacchesi S, Buchholz UJ, et al. The two major human metapneumovirus genetic lineages are highly related antigenically, and the fusion (F) protein is a major contributor to this antigenic relatedness. J Virol 2004;78:6927–37.

[8] Boivin G, Abed Y, Pelletier G, et al. Virological features and clinical manifestations associated with human metapneumovirus: a new paramyxovirus responsible for acute respiratory-tract infections in all age groups. J Infect Dis 2002;186:1330–4.

[9] Bastien N, Ward D, Van Caeseele P, et al. Human metapneumovirus infection in the Canadian population. J Clin Microbiol 2003;41:4642–6.

[10] van den Hoogen BG, van Doornum GJ, Fockens JC, et al. Prevalence and clinical symptoms of human metapneumovirus infection in hospitalized patients. J Infect Dis 2003;188:1571–7.

[11] Peiris JS, Tang WH, Chan KH, et al. Children with respiratory disease associated with metapneumovirus in Hong Kong. Emerg Infect Dis 2003;9:628–33.

[12] Boivin G, De Serres G, Cote S, et al. Human metapneumovirus infections in hospitalized children. Emerg Infect Dis 2003;9:634–40.

[13] Freymouth F, Vabret A, Legrand L, et al. Presence of the new human metapneumovirus in French children with bronchiolitis. Pediatr Infect Dis J 2003;22:92–4.

[14] Maggi F, Pifferi M, Vatteroni M, et al. Human metapneumovirus associated with respiratory tract infections in a 3-year study of nasal swabs from infants in Italy. J Clin Microbiol 2003;41:2987–91.

[15] Viazov S, Ratjen F, Scheidhauer R, Fiedler M, Roggendorf M. High prevalence of human metapneumovirus infection in young children and genetic heterogeneity of the viral isolates. J Clin Microbiol 2003;41:3043–5.

[16] Thanasugarn W, Samransamruajkit R, Vanapongtipagorn P, et al. Human metapneumovirus infection in Thai children. Scand J Infect Dis 2003;35:754–6.

[17] IJpma FF, Beekhuis D, Cotton MF, et al. Human metapneumovirus infection in hospital referred South African children. J Med Virol 2004;73:486–93.

[18] Galiano M, Videla C, Puch SS, Martinez A, Echavarria M, Carballal G. Evidence of human metapneumovirus in children in Argentina. J Med Virol 2004;72:299–303.

[19] Ebihara T, Endo R, Kikuta H, et al. Human metapneumovirus infection in Japanese children. J Clin Microbiol 2004;42:126–32.

[20] Cuevas LE, Nasser AM, Dove W, Gurgel RQ, Greensill J, Hart CA. Human metapneumovirus and respiratory syncytial virus, Brazil. Emerg Infect Dis 2003;9:1626–8.

[21] Zhu RN, Qian Y, Deng J, et al. Human metapneumovirus may associate with acute respiratory infections in hospitalized pediatric patients in Beijing, China. Zhonghua Er Ke Za Zhi 2003;41:441–4.

[22] Esper F, Martinello RA, Boucher D, et al. A 1-year experience with human metapneumovirus in children aged <5 years. J Infect Dis 2004;189:1388–96.

[23] Dollner H, Risnes K, Radtke A, Nordbo SA. An outbreak of human metapneumovirus infection in Norwegian children. Pediatr Infect Dis J 2004;23:436–40.

[24] McAdam AJ, Hasenbein ME, Feldman HA, et al. Human metapneumovirus in children tested at a tertiary-care hospital. J Infect Dis 2004;190:20–6.

[25] Mullins JA, Erdman DD, Weinberg GA, et al. Human metapneumovirus infection among children hospitalized with acute respiratory illness. Emerg Infect Dis 2004;10: 700–5.

[26] Bosis S, Esposito S, Niesters HG, Crovari P, Osterhaus AD, Principi N. Impact of human metapneumovirus in childhood: comparison with respiratory syncytial virus and influenza viruses. J Med Virol 2005;75:101–4.

[27] Bach N, Cuvillon D, Brouard J, et al. Acute respiratory tract infections due to a human metapneumovirus in children: descriptive study and comparison with respiratory syncytial virus infections. Arch Pediatr 2004;11:212–5.

[28] Rawlinson WD, Waliuzzaman Z, Carter IW, Belessis YC, Gilbert KM, Morton JR. Asthma exacerbations in children associated with rhinovirus but not human metapneumovirus infection. J Infect Dis 2003;187:1314–8.

[29] Jartti T, van den Hoogen B, Garofalo RP, Osterhaus AD, Ruuskanen O. Metapneumovirus and acute wheezing in children. Lancet 2002;360:1393–4.

[30] Laham FR, Israele V, Casellas JM, et al. Differential production of inflammatory cytokines in primary infection with human metapneumovirus and with other common respiratory viruses of infancy. J Infect Dis 2004;189:2047–56.

[31] Cane PA, van den Hoogen BG, Chakrabarti S, Fegan CD, Osterhaus AD. Human metapneumovirus in a haematopoietic stem cell transplant recipient with fatal lower respiratory tract disease. Bone Marrow Transplant 2003;31:309–10.

[32] Pelletier G, Dery P, Abed Y, Boivin G. Respiratory tract reinfections by the new human metapneumovirus in an immunocompromised child. Emerg Infect Dis 2002;8:976–8.

[33] Madhi SA, Ludewick H, Abed Y, Klugman KP, Boivin G. Human metapneumovirus-associated lower respiratory tract infections among hospitalized human immunodeficiency virus type 1 (HIV-1)-infected and HIV-1-uninfected African infants. Clin Infect Dis 2003;37: 1705–10.

[34] Garcia Garcia ML, Calvo Rey C, Martin del Valle F, et al. Respiratory infections due to metapneumovirus in hospitalized infants. An Pediatr (Barc) 2004;61:213–8.

[35] Konig B, Konig W, Arnold R, Werchau H, Ihorst G, Forster J. Prospective study of human metapneumovirus infection in children less than 3 years of age. J Clin Microbiol 2004;42: 4632–5.

[36] Greensill J, McNamara PS, Dove W, Flanagan B, Smyth RL, Hart CA. Human metapneumovirus in severe respiratory syncytial virus bronchiolitis. Emerg Infect Dis 2003;9:372–5.

[37] Semple MG, Cowell A, Dove W, et al. Dual infection of infants by human metapneumovirus and human respiratory syncytial virus is strongly associated with severe bronchiolitis. J Infect Dis 2005;191:382–6.

[38] Lazar I, Weibel C, Dziura J, Ferguson D, Landry ML, Kahn JS. Human metapneumovirus and severity of respiratory syncytial virus disease. Emerg Infect Dis 2004;10:1318–20.

[39] Monto AS. Medical reviews: coronaviruses. Yale J Biol Med 1974;47:234–51.

[40] McIntosh K, Chao RK, Krause HE, Wasil R, Mocega HE, Mufson MA. Coronavirus infection in acute lower respiratory tract disease of infants. J Infect Dis 1974;130:502–7.

[41] Kaye HS, Marsh HB, Dowdle WR. Seroepidemiologic survey of coronavirus (strain OC 43) related infections in a children's population. Am J Epidemiol 1971;94:43–9.

[42] Isaacs D, Flowers D, Clarke JR, Valman HB, MacNaughton MR. Epidemiology of coronavirus respiratory infections. Arch Dis Child 1983;58:500–3.

[43] Sizun J, Soupre D, Legrand MC, et al. Neonatal nosocomial respiratory infection with coronavirus: a prospective study in a neonatal intensive care unit. Acta Paediatr 1995;84: 617–20.

[44] Sizun J, Soupre D, Legrand MC, Giroux JD, Rubio S, Chastel C, et al. [Pathogen role of coronavirus in pediatric intensive care: retrospective analysis of 19 positive samples with indirect immunofluorescence]. Arch Pediatr 1994;1:477–80.

[45] Macnaughton MR, Flowers D, Isaacs D. Diagnosis of human coronavirus infections in children using enzyme-linked immunosorbent assay. J Med Virol 1983;11:319–25.

[46] Sizun J, Soupre D, Giroux JD, et al. Nasal colonization with coronavirus and apnea of the premature newborn. Acta Paediatr 1993;82:238.

[47] Gagneur A, Sizun J, Vallet S, Legr MC, Picard B, Talbot PJ. Coronavirus-related nosocomial viral respiratory infections in a neonatal and paediatric intensive care unit: a prospective study. J Hosp Infect 2002;51:59–64.

[48] Peiris JS, Lai ST, Poon LL, Guan Y, Yam LY, Lim W. Coronavirus as a possible cause of severe acute respiratory syndrome. Lancet 2003;361:1319–25.

[49] Ksiazek TG, Erdman D, Goldsmith CS, et al. A novel coronavirus associated with severe acute respiratory syndrome. N Engl J Med 2003;348:1953–66.

[50] Drosten C, Gunther S, Preiser W, et al. Identification of a novel coronavirus in patients with severe acute respiratory syndrome. N Engl J Med 2003;348:1967–76.

[51] Guan Y, Zheng BJ, He YQ, et al. Isolation and characterization of viruses related to SARS coronavirus from animals in southern China. Science 2003;302:276–8.

[52] World Health Organization. Summary of probable SARS cases with onset of illness from 1 November 2002 to 31 July 2003. Available at: http://www.who.int/csr/sars/country/table2004_04_21/en/. Accessed February 28, 2005.

[53] Hon KL, Leung CW, Cheng WT, et al. Clinical presentations and outcome of severe acute respiratory syndrome in children. Lancet 2003;361:1701–3.

[54] Chiu WK, Cheung PC, Ng KL, et al. Severe acute respiratory syndrome in children: experience in a regional hospital in Hong Kong. Pediatr Crit Care Med 2003;4:279–83.

[55] Leung CW, Kwan YW, Ko PW, et al. Severe acute respiratory syndrome among children. Pediatrics 2004;113:e535–43.

[56] Li AM, Chan CH, Chan DF. Long-term sequelae of SARS in children. Paediatr Respir Rev 2004;5:296–9.

[57] Shek CC, Ng PC, Fung GP, et al. Infants born to mothers with severe acute respiratory syndrome. Pediatrics 2003;112:e254.

[58] van der Hoek L, Pyrc K, Jebbink MF, et al. Identification of a new human coronavirus. Nat Med 2004;10:368–73.

[59] Fouchier RA, Hartwig NG, Bestebroer TM, et al. A previously undescribed coronavirus associated with respiratory disease in humans. Proc Natl Acad Sci U S A 2004;101:6212–6.

[60] Bastien N, Anderson K, Hart L, et al. Human coronavirus NL63 infection in Canada. J Infect Dis 2005;191:503–6.

[61] Esper F, Weibel C, Ferguson D, Landry ML, Kahn JS. Evidence of a novel human coronavirus that is associated with respiratory tract disease in infants and young children. J Infect Dis 2005;191:492–8.

[62] Neuzil KM, Mellen BG, Wright PF, Mitchel EF Jr, Griffin MR. The effect of influenza on hospitalizations, outpatient visits, and courses of antibiotics in children. N Engl J Med 2000; 342:225–31.

[63] Neuzil KM, Zhu Y, Griffin MR, et al. Burden of interpandemic influenza in children younger than 5 years: a 25-year prospective study. J Infect Dis 2002;185:147–52.

[64] Claas EC, Kawaoka Y, de Jong JC, Masurel N, Webster RG. Infection of children with avian-human reassortant influenza virus from pigs in Europe. Virology 1994;204:453–7.

[65] Subbarao K, Klimov A, Katz J, et al. Characterization of an avian influenza A (H5N1) virus isolated from a child with a fatal respiratory illness. Science 1998;279:393–6.

[66] Yuen KY, Chan PK, Peiris M, et al. Clinical features and rapid viral diagnosis of human disease associated with avian influenza A H5N1 virus. Lancet 1998;351:467–71.

[67] Peiris JSM, Yu WC, Leung CW, et al. Re-emergence of fatal human influenza A subtype H5N1 disease. Lancet 2004;363:617–9.

[68] Peiris M, Leung CW, Chan KH, et al. Human infection with influenza H9N2. Lancet 1999; 354:916–7.
[69] Centers for Disease Control and Prevention (CDC). Cases of influenza A (H5N1)—Thailand, 2004. MMWR Morb Mortal Wkly Rep 2004;53:100–3.
[70] Tran TH, Nguyen TL, Nguyen TD, et al. Avian influenza A (H5N1) in 10 patients in Vietnam. N Engl J Med 2004;350:1179–88.
[71] de Jong MD, Bach VC, Phan TQ, et al. Fatal avian influenza A (H5N1) in a child presenting with diarrhea followed by coma. N Engl J Med 2005;352:686–91.
[72] Murray K, Selleck P, Hooper P, et al. A morbillivirus that caused fatal disease in horses and humans: infection of humans and horses by a newly described morbillivirus. Science 1995; 268:94–7.
[73] Goh KJ, Tan CT, Chew NK, et al. Clinical features of Nipah virus encephalitis among pig farmers in Malaysia. N Engl J Med 2000;342:1229–35.
[74] Hsu VP, Hossain MJ, Parashar UD, et al. Nipah virus encephalitis reemergence, Bangladesh. Emerg Infect Dis 2004;10:2082–7.

ELSEVIER
SAUNDERS

INFECTIOUS
DISEASE CLINICS
OF NORTH AMERICA

Infect Dis Clin N Am 19 (2005) 585–602

Acute Diarrheal Disease in Children: Epidemiology, Prevention, and Treatment

Penelope H. Dennehy, MD[a,b,*]

[a]*Division of Pediatric Infectious Diseases, Rhode Island Hospital, 593 Eddy Street, Providence, RI 02903, USA*

[b]*Department of Pediatrics, Brown Medical School, Providence, RI 02903, USA*

Diarrhea is one of the most common causes of morbidity and mortality in children worldwide. Acute diarrhea accounts for 2 to 3 million deaths per year with most occurring in young children in developing countries [1]. In the United States, 220,000 children younger than 5 years of age are hospitalized each year with gastroenteritis accounting for approximately 9% of all hospitalizations in this age group [2]. The incidence of diarrhea in children younger than 3 years of age has been estimated to be 1.3 to 2.3 episodes per child per year; rates in children attending daycare centers are higher [3]. Hospitalization and outpatient care for pediatric diarrhea results in direct costs of more than $2 billion per year [4,5].

The causes of acute diarrhea in children vary with the location, time of year, and population studied. There is increasing recognition of a widening array of enteric pathogens associated with diarrheal disease. Agents such as enterohemorrhagic *Escherichia coli* (EHEC), *Salmonella, Shigella, Cryptosporidium, Giardia, Campylobacter jejuni, Clostridium difficile,* rotaviruses, caliciviruses, and other enteric viruses are among the pathogens that cause acute gastroenteritis in the United States (Table 1). Many of these organisms are transmitted easily through food or water or from one person to another, and some are devastating to individuals with compromised immune systems. Adequate fluid and electrolyte replacement and maintenance are key to managing diarrheal illnesses. Thorough clinical and epidemiologic evaluation is needed to define the severity and type of illness, exposures, and whether the

* Division of Pediatric Infectious Diseases, Rhode Island Hospital, 593 Eddy Street, Providence, RI 02903, USA.

E-mail address: pdennehy@lifespan.org

doi:10.1016/j.idc.2005.05.003 ***id.theclinics.com***

Table 1
Infectious causes of acute diarrhea in children in the United States

Viral	Bacterial	Parasitic
Rotavirus	*Campylobacter*	*Giardia intestinalis*
Calicivirus	*Salmonella*	*Cryptosporidium parvum*
Astrovirus	*Escherichia coli* O157:H7	
Enteric adenovirus	*Shigella*	
	Clostridium difficile	
	Yersinia enterocolitica	

patient is immunocompromised to direct the performance of selective diagnostic cultures, toxin testing, parasite studies, and the administration of antimicrobial therapy. Increasing numbers of enteric bacterial pathogens resistant to antimicrobial agents complicate therapy further.

Viral causes of diarrhea

Viruses are most common pathogens causing diarrheal illness in the United States in all age groups [6]. Rotaviruses and noroviruses are the most frequently observed pathogens. Other viral pathogens that have been observed in the stools of children with diarrhea include astroviruses and enteric adenoviruses.

Rotavirus infections

Rotaviruses are segmented, double-stranded RNA viruses with at least seven distinct antigenic groups (A through G). Group A viruses are the major cause of rotavirus diarrhea worldwide. Serotyping is based on the VP7 glycoprotein (G) and VP4 protease-cleaved hemagglutinin (P). To date, 15 G types and 20 P types have been described for group A rotaviruses, and at least 10 G types and 8 P types cause human infections. G types 1 through 4 and 9 and P types 1A and 1B are most common [7]. In recent years, previously uncommon G types have increased in frequency, especially G5, G6, G8, and G10 [8]. Monitoring the frequency of G and P antigenic types is important to target the appropriate antigens for vaccine development.

Rotavirus infection causes approximately 600,000 to 875,000 deaths annually worldwide and is responsible for 6% of all deaths in children younger than 5 years of age [9]. The burden of disease is most severe in developing countries. In the United States, rotavirus infection is the leading cause of hospitalization for gastroenteritis in infants and young children and is responsible for 600,000 physician visits, 50,000 hospitalizations, and at least 20 deaths each year [10].

Transmission is presumed to be by the fecal-oral route. Rotavirus is present in high titers in stools of infected patients with diarrhea and in stool before the onset of diarrhea. Rotavirus shedding can persist for 21 days after the onset of symptoms in immunocompetent hosts. Virus can be found on toys and hard surfaces in daycare centers, indicating that fomites may serve as a mechanism of transmission [11]. Spread within families and institutions is common. Rotavirus is the most common cause of hospital-acquired diarrhea in children and is an important cause of acute gastroenteritis in children attending daycare centers.

In temperate climates, disease is most prevalent during the cooler months. Seasonal patterns in tropical climates are less pronounced, but disease is more common during the drier, cooler months.

Virtually all children are infected by 3 years of age. Rotavirus gastroenteritis most commonly occurs in infants and children 4 to 24 months old. Infections during the first 3 months of life and reinfections among older children are more likely to be asymptomatic. Thirty percent to 50% of adult contacts of infected infants become infected, although most are asymptomatic.

Rotavirus illness begins with acute onset of fever and vomiting followed by watery diarrhea [12]. Typically there are 10 to 20 bowel movements per day. Symptoms generally persist for 3 to 8 days. Dehydration and electrolyte disturbances are the major sequelae of rotavirus infection and occur most often in the youngest children. Patients with immunodeficiency, including those with HIV, solid-organ or bone marrow transplantation, and natural killer cell deficiency, may have more severe or prolonged diarrhea [13–17]. A large study in Malawian children found no difference, however, in clinical disease between HIV-infected and noninfected patients [18].

Enzyme immunoassay and latex agglutination assays for group A rotavirus antigen detection in stool are available commercially. Virus also can be identified in stool by electron microscopy and by reverse transcriptase polymerase chain reaction.

No specific antiviral therapy is available. Oral or parenteral fluids are given to prevent and correct dehydration [19]. A vaccine to prevent rotavirus infection and disease is not available commercially. The rhesus rotavirus tetravalent vaccine (RotaShield) licensed by the US Food and Drug Administration in August 1998 and incorporated into the 1999 routine immunization schedule is no longer recommended for use because of the association of this vaccine with intussusception [20] This product was withdrawn voluntarily from the market in October 1999. A monovalent live attenuated human rotavirus vaccine was licensed in Mexico [21]. A second vaccine, a pentavalent human-bovine reassortant vaccine, has just completed clinical trials and is expected to be licensed within the next several years [22].

Calicivirus infections

Caliciviruses are a family of single-stranded, nonenveloped RNA viruses. The two recognized genera that cause diarrheal disease in humans are noroviruses (Norwalk-like viruses) and sapoviruses (Sapporo-like viruses) [23]. Human caliciviruses have a worldwide distribution, with multiple antigenic types circulating simultaneously in the same region. Noroviruses and sapoviruses are major causes of sporadic cases of gastroenteritis requiring hospitalization. Most sporadic calicivirus infections have been detected in children younger than 4 years of age [24].

Noroviruses are the most common cause of outbreaks of nonbacterial gastroenteritis, and it is estimated that they are responsible for 68% to 80% of all outbreaks of gastroenteritis in industrialized countries. The Centers for Disease Control and Prevention estimates that at least 50% of all food-borne outbreaks of gastroenteritis can be attributed to noroviruses. Among the 232 outbreaks of norovirus illness reported to the Centers for Disease Control from July 1997 to June 2000, 57% were food-borne [25]. In this study, common settings for outbreaks include restaurants and catered meals, nursing homes, schools, and vacation settings or cruise ships.

Noroviruses are transmitted primarily through the fecal-oral route, either by consumption of contaminated food or water or by direct person-to-person spread. Environmental contamination also may act as a source of infection. Good evidence exists for transmission secondary to aerosolization of vomitus that presumably results in droplets contaminating surfaces or entering the oral mucosa and being swallowed [26,27]. Noroviruses are highly contagious. An inoculum of 10 viral particles may be sufficient to infect an individual.

Norovirus infection usually presents with acute onset of vomiting, watery nonbloody diarrhea with abdominal cramps, and nausea. Low-grade fever also occasionally occurs. Vomiting is more common in children. Dehydration is the most common complication, especially among young and elderly patients. Symptoms usually last 24 to 60 hours.

Diagnosis of norovirus illness in outbreaks has improved with the increasing use of reverse transcriptase polymerase chain reaction [28]. Currently, 27 state public health laboratories have the capability to test for noroviruses by reverse transcriptase polymerase chain reaction. This test can be used to test stool and emesis samples and to detect the presence of noroviruses on environmental swabs.

No specific therapy exists for calicivirus gastroenteritis. Symptomatic therapy consists of replacing fluid losses and correcting electrolyte disturbances through oral and intravenous fluid administration.

Astrovirus infections

Astroviruses are nonenveloped, single-stranded RNA viruses with a characteristic starlike appearance by electron microscopy. Eight human antigenic types are known. Astroviruses have a worldwide distribution. Multiple antigenic types co-circulate in the same region [29].

Astroviruses are increasingly recognized as significant gastrointestinal pathogens. These viruses have been detected in 10% of sporadic cases of nonbacterial gastroenteritis among young children [30]. Astrovirus infections occur primarily in children younger than 4 years of age and have a seasonal peak in the winter. Transmission is person to person via the fecal-oral route. Outbreaks often occur in closed populations, and attack rates are high in hospitalized children and in children in daycare centers. Viral shedding lasts for an average of 5 days after onset of symptoms. Children may shed asymptomatically for several weeks after the illness, and persistent shedding may occur in immunocompromised hosts [31].

Illness caused by astroviruses is characterized by abdominal pain, diarrhea, vomiting, nausea, fever, and malaise. In the immunocompetent host, disease is self-limited, lasting 5 to 6 days on average. Asymptomatic infections are common.

Commercial tests for diagnosis of astrovirus infection are not available in the United States. Enzyme immunoassays are available in many other countries.

Treatment of astrovirus infection is supportive. Rehydration with oral or intravenous fluid and electrolyte solution is the mainstay of therapy.

Enteric adenovirus infections

Adenoviruses are double-stranded, nonenveloped DNA viruses; at least 51 distinct serotypes cause human infections. Serotypes 40, 41, and, to a lesser extent, 31 are associated with gastroenteritis. Enteric adenoviral disease occurs throughout the year and primarily affects children younger than 4 years of age. Adenovirus infections are most communicable during the first few days of an acute illness, but persistent and intermittent shedding for longer periods is common. Transmission is via the fecal-oral route. Asymptomatic infections are common, and reinfections can occur.

The clinical picture is similar to that of rotavirus. In contrast to the nonenteric adenoviruses, high fevers and respiratory symptoms are rare. Disease can be persistent and severe in the immunocompromised host. Specific adenovirus colitis has been reported in HIV-infected patients [32].

The preferred method for diagnosis of enteric adenovirus infection is antigen detection by immunoassay techniques. Enteric adenovirus types 40 and 41 usually cannot be isolated in standard cell cultures.

Treatment of enteric adenovirus infection is supportive. Rehydration with oral or intravenous fluid and electrolyte solution is the mainstay of therapy.

Bacterial causes of diarrhea

In developed countries, bacterial pathogens account for 2% to 10% of cases of diarrhea [33]. *Campylobacter, Salmonella, Shigella,* and EHEC account for most cases in the United States. *Yersinia enterocolitica, Vibrio* species including *Vibrio cholerae* and non-01 cholera, *Aeromonas,* and *Plesiomonas* are unusual sources of diarrhea in developed countries.

The clinical presentation of bacterial gastroenteritis overlaps with viral disease, and the two can be indistinguishable clinically. A few clinical and laboratory clues make a bacterial cause more likely, however. High fevers, shaking chills, and blood in the stools are unusual in acute viral gastroenteritis. The presence of leukocytes in a stool specimen is helpful for discriminating bacterial gastroenteritis from viral disease.

Campylobacter *infections*

Campylobacter species are motile, comma-shaped, gram-negative bacilli. *Campylobacter jejuni* and *Campylobacter coli* are the most common species isolated from patients with diarrhea and are the major organisms reported by the Foodborne Diseases Active Surveillance Network (FoodNet) [34]. *Campylobacter* is found in the gastrointestinal tract of domestic and wild birds and animals. Poultry carcasses usually are contaminated. Many farm animals can harbor the organism, and pets, especially young animals, are potential sources. Transmission of *Campylobacter* occurs by ingestion of contaminated food or by direct contact with fecal material from infected animals or people [35]. Improperly cooked poultry, untreated water, and unpasteurized milk have been the main vehicles of transmission. Person-to-person spread occurs occasionally, particularly from very young children, and outbreaks of diarrhea in daycare centers have been reported infrequently. Shedding of *Campylobacter* organisms usually lasts 2 to 3 weeks.

Campylobacter infections present with a wide clinical spectrum ranging from mild diarrhea to dysentery [36]. Symptoms most commonly seen include diarrhea, abdominal pain, malaise, and fever. In neonates and young infants, bloody diarrhea without fever may be the only manifestation of infection. Abdominal pain can mimic appendicitis. Mild infection lasts 1 or 2 days and resembles viral gastroenteritis. Most patients recover in less than 1 week, but 20% relapse or have a prolonged illness [37]. Severe or persistent infection can mimic acute inflammatory bowel disease [38]. *Campylobacter jejuni* and *Campylobacter coli* can be cultured from feces, but require selective media.

Most cases of *Campylobacter* infection are self-limited and do not require antibiotic therapy. Treatment may be indicated in more severe cases because erythromycin and azithromycin shorten the duration of illness and prevent relapse when given early [39]. Treatment usually eradicates the organism from stool within 2 or 3 days. Doxycycline, for children 8 years old or older, is an alternative agent. Fluoroquinolones are effective, but are not licensed for people younger than 18 years old. If antimicrobial therapy is given, the recommended duration is 5 to 7 days.

Salmonella *infections*

Salmonella organisms are gram-negative bacilli that belong to the Enterobacteriaceae family. The principal reservoirs for nontyphoidal *Salmonella* organisms are animals, including poultry, livestock, reptiles, and pets. The major vehicles of transmission are foods of animal origin, including poultry, beef, fish, eggs, and dairy products [40]. Many other foods, including fruits, vegetables, and bakery products, have been implicated in outbreaks. These foods usually are contaminated by contact with an animal product or, occasionally, an infected human. Other modes of transmission include ingestion of contaminated water and contact with infected reptiles [41].

Age-specific attack rates for *Salmonella* infection are highest in people younger than 4 years of age, with a peak during the first months of life. Rates of invasive infections and mortality are higher in infants; elderly people; and people with immunosuppressive conditions, hemoglobinopathies, malignant neoplasms, and AIDS [42]. Most reported cases are sporadic, but widespread outbreaks have been reported. From 1996 through 2000, *Salmonella* was second to *Campylobacter* as the cause of laboratory-confirmed cases of enteric disease as reported by the FoodNet [34].

The risk of transmission exists as long as fecal shedding is present. Twelve weeks after infection, 45% of children younger than 5 years of age shed *Salmonella* compared with 5% of older children and adults. Antimicrobial therapy can prolong shedding. Approximately 1% of patients continue to shed *Salmonella* for more than 1 year and are chronic carriers.

Infection with nontyphoidal *Salmonella* causes a spectrum of illness ranging from asymptomatic carriage, gastroenteritis, and bacteremia to focal infections, such as meningitis and osteomyelitis. The most common illness associated with nontyphoidal *Salmonella* is gastroenteritis. Diarrhea, abdominal cramps and tenderness, and fever are common manifestations. The site of infection usually is the small intestine, but colitis can occur. Sustained or intermittent bacteremia can occur, and focal infections are recognized in 10% of patients with bacteremia resulting from *Salmonella* infection. Isolation of *Salmonella* organisms from cultures of stool, blood, urine, and material from foci of infection is diagnostic.

Antimicrobial therapy usually is not indicated for patients with uncomplicated, noninvasive *Salmonella* gastroenteritis because therapy does not shorten the duration of disease and may prolong the duration of carriage. Although of unproven benefit, antimicrobial therapy is recommended for gastroenteritis caused by *Salmonella* species in patients with an increased risk of invasive disease, including infants younger than 3 months of age and patients with chronic gastrointestinal tract disease, malignant neoplasms, hemoglobinopathies, HIV infection or other immunosuppressive illnesses or therapies, or severe colitis [39]. Ampicillin, amoxicillin, trimethoprim-sulfamethoxazole, cefotaxime, and ceftriaxone are recommended for susceptible strains in patients for whom therapy is indicated [39]. Strains acquired in developing countries often exhibit resistance to many antimicrobial agents, but usually are susceptible to ceftriaxone or cefotaxime and to fluoroquinolones.

Shigella *infections*

Shigella species are aerobic, gram-negative bacilli in the family Enterobacteriaceae. Four species have been identified. Among *Shigella* isolates reported in the United States from 1989 to 2003, 87.9% were *S sonnei,* 11% were *S flexneri,* 0.8% were *S boydii,* and 0.2% were *S dysenteriae. Shigella dysenteriae* is rare in the United States, but is endemic in rural Africa and the Indian subcontinent.

Humans are the natural host for *Shigella.* The primary mode of transmission is fecal-oral. Children 5 years of age or younger in daycare settings, their caregivers, and other people living in crowded conditions are at increased risk of infection. Travel to developing countries with inadequate sanitation may place the traveler at risk of infection. Ingestion of 10 to 200 organisms is sufficient for infection to occur depending on the *Shigella* species. Predominant modes of transmission include person-to-person contact, contact with a contaminated inanimate object, ingestion of contaminated food and water, and sexual contact. Houseflies also may be vectors through physical transport of infected feces [43]. Fecal shedding usually lasts for only a few weeks after illness. Chronic carriage of *Shigella* is rare.

Shigella primarily infect the large intestine, causing clinical manifestations that range from watery or loose stools with minimal or no constitutional symptoms to more severe symptoms, including fever, abdominal cramps or tenderness, tenesmus, and mucoid stools with or without blood. Clinical presentations vary with *Shigella* species. *S sonnei* infection usually produces watery diarrhea, whereas *S flexneri, S boydii,* and *S dysenteriae* infections typically cause bloody diarrhea and severe systemic symptoms. Rare complications include bacteremia, hemolytic uremic syndrome (HUS) (after *S dysenteriae* type 1 infection), toxic megacolon and perforation, and toxic encephalopathy (ekiri).

Cultures of feces or rectal swab specimens are diagnostic, but lack sensitivity. The presence of fecal leukocytes suggests colitis. Although bacteremia is rare, blood should be cultured in severely ill, immunocompromised, or malnourished patients.

Most clinical infections with *S sonnei* are self-limited (48–72 hours) and do not require antimicrobial therapy. Antimicrobial therapy is effective, however, in shortening the duration of diarrhea and eradicating organisms from feces. Treatment is recommended for patients with severe disease, dysentery, or underlying immunosuppressive conditions. In mild disease, the primary indication for treatment is to prevent spread of the organism.

Antimicrobial susceptibility testing of clinical isolates is indicated because resistance to antimicrobial agents is common. Plasmid-mediated resistance has been identified in all *Shigella* species. In the United States, sentinel surveillance data in 2001 indicated that 80% of *S sonnei* were resistant to ampicillin, and 47% were resistant to trimethoprim-sulfamethoxazole.

For cases in which susceptibility is unknown or an ampicillin-resistant and trimethoprim-sulfamethoxazole–resistant strain is isolated, ceftriaxone, a fluoroquinolone (for patients >18 years old), or azithromycin may be given [39]. For susceptible strains, ampicillin and trimethoprim-sulfamethoxazole are effective. Amoxicillin is less effective because of its rapid absorption from the gastrointestinal tract. The oral route of therapy is recommended except for seriously ill patients. Antimicrobial therapy should be administered for 5 days. Antidiarrheal compounds that inhibit intestinal peristalsis are contraindicated because they may prolong the clinical and bacteriologic course of disease.

Diarrhea-associated Escherichia coli

At least five types of diarrhea-producing *E coli* strains have been identified. Clinical features of disease caused by each type are summarized in Table 2. Transmission of most diarrhea-associated *E coli* strains is from food or water contaminated with human or animal feces or from infected symptomatic people or carriers. The only *E coli* type that commonly causes diarrhea in the United States is EHEC, especially *E coli* O157:H7, which is shed in feces of cattle. EHEC can be transmitted by undercooked ground beef, contaminated water and produce, unpasteurized milk, and a wide variety of vehicles contaminated with bovine feces. Infections caused by *E coli* O157:H7 are detected sporadically or during outbreaks. Outbreaks have been linked to ground beef, petting zoos, contaminated apple cider, raw fruits and vegetables, salami, yogurt, drinking water, and ingestion of

Table 2
Classification of *Escherichia coli* associated with diarrhea

E coli type	Epidemiology	Type of diarrhea
Enterohemorrahgic	Hemorrhagic colitis and hemolytic uremic syndrome in all ages and postdiarrheal thrombotic thrombocytopenic purpura in adults	Bloody or nonbloody
Enteropathogenic	Acute and chronic endemic and epidemic diarrhea in infants	Watery
Enterotoxigenic	Infantile diarrhea in developing countries and traveler's diarrhea in all ages	Watery
Enteroinvasive	Diarrhea with fever in all ages	Bloody or nonbloody; dysentery
Enteroaggregative	Acute and chronic diarrhea in infants	Watery, occasionally bloody

water in recreational areas. The infectious dose is approximately 100 organisms, and person-to-person transmission is common during outbreaks.

EHEC strains are associated with diarrhea, hemorrhagic colitis, HUS, and postdiarrheal thrombotic thrombocytopenic purpura. Illness caused by EHEC often begins as nonbloody diarrhea, but usually progresses to diarrhea with visible or occult blood. Severe abdominal pain is typical; fever occurs in less than one third of cases. Severe infection can result in hemorrhagic colitis. HUS, defined as the triad of microangiopathic hemolytic anemia, thrombocytopenia, and acute renal dysfunction, is the most serious sequela of EHEC infection and seems to occur more frequently with *E coli* O157:H7 than other EHEC serotypes. HUS occurs in 8% of children with *E coli* O157:H7 diarrhea [44]. HUS usually develops in the 2 weeks after onset of diarrhea. Thrombotic thrombocytopenic purpura occurs in adults and is the same disease as postdiarrheal HUS. Non-EHEC types are associated with disease predominantly in developing countries, where food and water supplies commonly are contaminated, and facilities and supplies for hand hygiene are suboptimal. Enterotoxigenic *E coli* is the major cause of traveler's diarrhea.

Diagnosis of infection caused by diarrhea-associated *E coli* usually is difficult because most clinical laboratories cannot differentiate diarrhea-associated *E coli* strains from normal stool flora *E coli* strains. The exception is *E coli* O157:H7, which can be identified by using MacConkey agar base with sorbitol substituted for lactose. Approximately 90% of human intestinal *E coli* strains rapidly ferment sorbitol, whereas *E coli* O157:H7 strains do not. Sorbitol-negative *E coli* can be serotyped, using commercially available antisera, to determine whether they are O157:H7. For all patients with HUS, stool specimens should be cultured for *E coli* O157:H7 and, if results are negative, for other EHEC serotypes. When EHEC infection is considered, a stool culture should be obtained as early in the illness as possible.

Dehydration and electrolyte abnormalities should be corrected. Antimotility agents should not be administered to children with inflammatory or bloody diarrhea [45]. Careful follow-up of patients with hemorrhagic colitis, including complete blood cell count with smear, blood urea nitrogen, and creatinine concentrations, is recommended to detect changes suggesting HUS. If patients have no laboratory evidence of hemolysis, thrombocytopenia, or nephropathy 3 days after resolution of diarrhea, their risk of developing HUS is low.

Although some studies have suggested that children with hemorrhagic colitis caused by EHEC have a greater risk of developing HUS if treated with antimicrobial agents compared with children not treated with antimicrobial agents, a meta-analysis failed to confirm this increased risk or to show a benefit [46]. Most experts would not treat children with *E coli* O157:H7 enteritis with an antimicrobial agent because no benefit has been proven, and such treatment may increase the risk of HUS [39,45].

Clostridium difficile

C difficile is a spore-forming, obligately anaerobic, gram-positive bacillus. Disease is related to the action of the toxins produced by this organism. Although other toxins also exist, toxins A and B have been associated most strongly with human disease.

C difficile can be isolated from soil and commonly is present in the environment. *C difficile* is acquired from the environment or from stool of other colonized or infected persons by the fecal-oral route. Intestinal colonization rates in healthy neonates and young infants can be 50%, but usually are less than 5% in children older than 2 years of age and in adults. Hospitals, nursing homes, and daycare centers are major reservoirs for *C difficile*. Risk factors for disease are those that increase exposure to organisms, such as prolonged hospitalization, and those that diminish the barrier effect of the normal intestinal flora, allowing *C difficile* to proliferate and elaborate toxins in vivo. Penicillins, clindamycin, and cephalosporins are the antimicrobial drugs most commonly associated with *C difficile* colitis, but colitis has been associated with almost every antimicrobial agent. Although *C difficile* toxin rarely is recovered from stool specimens of asymptomatic adults, it may be recovered from stool specimens from neonates and infants who have no gastrointestinal tract illness. This finding confounds the interpretation of positive toxin assays in patients younger than 12 months of age.

Syndromes associated with infections include pseudomembranous colitis and antimicrobial-associated diarrhea. Pseudomembranous colitis is characterized by diarrhea, abdominal cramps, fever, systemic toxicity, abdominal tenderness, and passage of stools containing blood and mucus. Disease usually begins while the person is receiving antimicrobial therapy, but it can occur weeks after therapy is completed. In rare cases, the illness is not associated with antimicrobial therapy or hospitalization. Infection also may result only in mild diarrhea or asymptomatic carriage.

Stool should be tested for the presence of *C difficile* toxins to diagnose *C difficile* disease. Commercially available enzyme immunoassays detect toxins A and B, or an enzyme immunoassay for toxin A may be used in conjunction with cell culture cytotoxicity assay, the "gold standard" for toxin B detection. Latex agglutination tests should not be used. Symptomatic infants younger than 1 year of age should be investigated for causes of diarrhea other than *C difficile* because the carriage of *C difficile* is the rule rather than the exception in this age group, and the presence of *C difficile* toxin may not be responsible for clinical signs.

In patients in whom clinically significant diarrhea or colitis develops, antimicrobial therapy should be discontinued as soon as possible. Antimicrobial therapy for *C difficile* disease is indicated for patients with severe disease or in whom diarrhea persists after antimicrobial therapy is discontinued. Metronidazole is the drug of choice for the initial treatment of most patients with colitis [39]. Oral vancomycin is an alternative drug and is indicated for patients who do not respond to metronidazole. Antimicrobial agents usually are administered for at least 10 days. Forty percent of patients experience a relapse after discontinuing therapy, but the infection usually responds to a second course of the same treatment. Drugs that decrease intestinal motility should not be administered.

Parasitic causes of diarrhea

Parasitic causes of diarrhea are common in pediatric patients. In developed countries, parasites account for 1% to 8% of cases of diarrhea. *Giardia* and *Cryptosporidium* infections are the most common causes of disease in the United States. *Entamoeba histolytica* is a common cause of diarrhea and dysentery in developing countries.

Giardia intestinalis *infections*

Giardia intestinalis is a flagellated protozoan that has a worldwide distribution. It is also the most common parasite cause of diarrhea in the United States. *Giardia* exists in trophozoite and cyst forms; the infective form is the cyst. Infection is limited to the small intestine and biliary tract.

Humans are the principal reservoir of infection, but *Giardia* can infect dogs, cats, beavers, and other animals. These animals can contaminate water with feces containing cysts that are infectious for humans. People become infected directly (by hand-to-mouth transfer of cysts from feces of an infected person) or indirectly (by ingestion of fecally contaminated water or food). Most community-wide epidemics have resulted from a contaminated water supply. Epidemics resulting from person-to-person transmission occur in daycare centers and in institutions for people with developmental disabilities. Cyst excretion may last for many months. The disease is communicable for as long as the infected person excretes cysts.

Symptomatic infection causes a broad spectrum of clinical manifestations. Many people who become infected with *G intestinalis* remain asymptomatic. Most symptomatic patients have mild diarrhea. Abdominal bloating and cramping also are common. Children may experience a protracted, intermittent, often debilitating disease, which is characterized by passage of foul-smelling stools associated with flatulence, abdominal distention, and anorexia. Anorexia combined with malabsorption can lead to significant weight loss, failure to thrive, and anemia.

Identification of trophozoites or cysts in direct smear examination or immunofluorescence antibody testing of stool specimens or duodenal fluid is diagnostic. Direct microscopic identification of cysts or trophozoites in the stool requires three separate stool specimens to reach 95% sensitivity.

Metronidazole is the drug of choice for treating symptomatic giardiasis; a 5- to 7-day course of therapy has a cure rate of 80% to 95% [47].

Tinidazole, a nitroimidazole, has a cure rate of 90% to 100% after a single dose, but limited safety and efficacy data are available in children. Furazolidone is 72% to 100% effective when given for 7 to 10 days. Albendazole [48] and mebendazole have been shown to be as effective as metronidazole for treating giardiasis in children, and they have fewer adverse effects. A 3-day course of nitazoxanide oral suspension is as effective as metronidazole and has the advantage of treating multiple other intestinal parasites. If therapy fails, a course can be repeated with the same drug. Relapse is common in immunocompromised patients, who may require prolonged treatment. Asymptomatic carriers should not be treated except to prevent spread in situations where they are in close contact with immunocompromised patients.

Cryptosporidiosis

Cryptosporidium parvum is a spore-forming coccidian protozoan. Oocysts are excreted in feces and are the infectious form. *C parvum* has been found in a variety of hosts, including mammals, birds, and reptiles. Extensive waterborne outbreaks have been associated with contamination of municipal water and exposure to contaminated swimming pools. Transmission to humans can occur from farm livestock, particularly young animals including those found in petting zoos, or pets. Person-to-person transmission occurs and can cause outbreaks in daycare centers, with attack rates of 30% to 60% reported. *C parvum* also causes traveler's diarrhea.

Infection with *C parvum* generally produces a benign self-limited diarrhea, although prolonged loose stools in otherwise healthy children have been seen. Fever and vomiting are relatively common among children and often lead to a misdiagnosis of viral gastroenteritis. Infection can be asymptomatic. Patients who are immunodeficient, especially patients with HIV infection, may develop chronic severe diarrhea, resulting in malnutrition, dehydration, and death. In most people, shedding of *C parvum* stops within 2 weeks, but in a few, shedding continues for 2 months.

The detection of oocysts on microscopic examination of stool specimens is diagnostic. Routine laboratory examination of stool for ova and parasites does not detect *C parvum*. The sucrose flotation method or formalin-ethyl acetate method is used to concentrate oocysts in stool before staining with a modified Kinyoun acid-fast stain. Direct fluorescence antibody staining for oocysts in stool and an enzyme immunoassay for detecting antigen in stool are available commercially. Because shedding can be intermittent, at least three stool specimens collected on separate days should be examined before considering test results to be negative.

Supportive care with rehydration and adequate nutrition usually is all that is required for therapy. A 3-day course of nitazoxanide oral suspension has been licensed by the Food and Drug Administration for treatment of children with cryptosporidial diarrhea [47,49], In immunocompromised patients with cryptosporidiosis, oral administration of human immune globulin or bovine colostrum has been beneficial. In HIV-infected patients, antiretroviral therapy–associated improvement in CD4 cell count can improve the course of disease [49].

Management of diarrheal disease in children

Prevention

Prevention remains the most vital measure in managing diarrheal disease. Vaccines are not currently available for any of the diarrheal pathogens, making efforts to interrupt transmission of infection crucial. Important measures to prevent spread of enteric pathogens include proper sanitation methods for food processing and preparation, sanitary water supplies, pasteurization of milk, proper hand hygiene, sanitary sewage disposal, exclusion of infected people from handling food or providing health care, and exclusion of people with diarrhea from use of public recreational water (eg, swimming pools, lakes, ponds).

Eggs and other foods of animal origin should be cooked thoroughly. Raw eggs and food containing raw eggs should not be eaten. Washing hands after handling raw poultry, washing cutting boards and utensils with soap and water after contact with raw poultry, avoiding contact of fruits and vegetables with the juices of raw poultry, and thorough cooking of poultry are critical. Washing hands after contact with feces of dogs and cats, particularly stool of puppies and kittens with diarrhea, also is important. The most important procedure to minimize fecal-oral transmission in daycare centers is frequent hand hygiene measures combined with staff training and monitoring of staff procedures.

Oral rehydration therapy

The current mainstay of treatment of acute gastroenteritis consists of oral rehydration and early introduction of feedings [39,50]. Treatment of dehydration with the World Health Organization oral rehydration solution (ORS) has decreased substantially deaths from cholera and other diarrheal diseases in developing countries. In the United States, the absence of cholera and the generally high level of nutrition and generous total body sodium levels in children have led to development of a consensus of ORS containing less sodium. Both solutions have been shown to be safe and effective in treating dehydration associated with acute diarrhea.

Hydration status in children can be assessed on the basis of easily observed signs and symptoms. Children who are not thirsty and have moist mucous membranes, wet diapers, and tears are not dehydrated and do not require ORS. In the absence of dehydration, ORS should be used to replace ongoing stool losses only in severe cases in which the patient already has required rehydration and still has ongoing diarrhea.

Children who are severely dehydrated with changes in vital signs or mental status require emergency intravenous fluid resuscitation. Hypotension is a late manifestation of shock in children. Mental status, heart rate, and perfusion are better indicators of severe dehydration and incipient shock. After initial treatment with intravenous fluids, these children can be given oral rehydration.

Children who are mildly or moderately dehydrated should receive 50 to 100 mL/kg of ORS over 4 hours and should be re-evaluated often for changes in hydration status. Children who are vomiting generally tolerate ORS. ORS is contraindicated in a child who is obtunded or at risk for aspiration. When oral hydration therapy is complete, regular feeding should be resumed.

Early refeeding

Early refeeding is recommended in managing acute gastroenteritis because luminal contents are a known growth factor for enterocytes and help facilitate mucosal repair after injury. Introducing a regular diet within a few hours of rehydration or continuing the diet during diarrhea without dehydration has been shown to shorten the duration of the disease. Early refeeding has not been associated with increased morbidity, such as electrolyte disturbance or a need for intravenous therapy.

Almost all infants with acute gastroenteritis can tolerate breastfeeding. For formula-fed infants, diluted formula does not provide any benefit over full-strength formula. Infants with the most severe diarrhea may require lactose-free formula until mucosal recovery is complete at around 2 weeks. Older children can consume a regular age-appropriate diet. No data suggest that a diet consisting of only bananas, rice, applesauce, and toast (the BRAT diet) speeds recovery from diarrheal illnesses. Lactose restriction is not usually necessary.

Future improvements in diarrhea management and prevention

Measures to decrease the duration of diarrheal illnesses are needed. Research on developing new ORS that would decrease the volume of loose stools is ongoing. Probiotics and other natural products that may have an effect on shortening episodes of acute infectious diarrhea are being studied [51,52]. Finally, prevention of diarrheal diseases by immunization is desirable. Vaccines to prevent rotavirus, shigella, cholera, and enterotoxigenic *E coli* infection are in clinical trials [53].

References

[1] Kosek M, Bern C, Guerrant RL. The global burden of diarrhoeal disease, as estimated from studies published between 1992 and 2000. Bull World Health Organ 2003;81:197–204.

[2] Glass RI, Kilgore PE, Holman RC, et al. The epidemiology of rotavirus diarrhea in the United States: surveillance and estimates of disease burden. J Infect Dis 1996;174(Suppl 1): S5–11.
[3] Guerrant RL, Hughes JM, Lima NL, Crane J. Diarrhea in developed and developing countries: magnitude, special settings, and etiologies. Rev Infect Dis 1990;12(Suppl 1): S41–50.
[4] Tucker AW, Haddix AC, Bresee JS, Holman RC, Parashar UD, Glass RI. Cost-effectiveness analysis of a rotavirus immunization program for the United States. JAMA 1998;279: 1371–6.
[5] Matson DO, Estes MK. Impact of rotavirus infection at a large pediatric hospital. J Infect Dis 1990;162:598–604.
[6] Wilhelmi I, Roman E, Sanchez-Fauquier A. Viruses causing gastroenteritis. Clin Microbiol Infect 2003;9:247–62.
[7] Griffin DD, Kirkwood CD, Parashar UD, et al. Surveillance of rotavirus strains in the United States: identification of unusual strains. The National Rotavirus Strain Surveillance System collaborating laboratories. J Clin Microbiol 2000;38:2784–7.
[8] Gentsch JR, Woods PA, Ramachandran M, et al. Review of G and P typing results from a global collection of rotavirus strains: implications for vaccine development. J Infect Dis 1996;174(Suppl 1):S30–6.
[9] Parashar UD, Hummelman EG, Bresee JS, Miller MA, Glass RI. Global illness and deaths caused by rotavirus disease in children. Emerg Infect Dis 2003;9:565–72.
[10] Ho MS, Glass RI, Pinsky PF, Anderson LJ. Rotavirus as a cause of diarrheal morbidity and mortality in the United States. J Infect Dis 1988;158:1112–6.
[11] Wilde J, Van R, Pickering L, Eiden J, Yolken R. Detection of rotaviruses in the day care environment by reverse transcriptase polymerase chain reaction. J Infect Dis 1992;166: 507–11.
[12] Staat MA, Azimi PH, Berke T, et al. Clinical presentations of rotavirus infection among hospitalized children. Pediatr Infect Dis J 2002;21:221–7.
[13] Thea DM, Glass R, Grohmann GS, et al. Prevalence of enteric viruses among hospital patients with AIDS in Kinshasa, Zaire. Trans R Soc Trop Med Hyg 1993;87:263–6.
[14] Thomas PD, Pollok RC, Gazzard BG. Enteric viral infections as a cause of diarrhoea in the acquired immunodeficiency syndrome. HIV Med 1999;1:19–24.
[15] Ziring D, Tran R, Edelstein S, et al. Infectious enteritis after intestinal transplantation: incidence, timing, and outcome. Transplantation 2005;79:702–9.
[16] Kang G, Srivastava A, Pulimood AB, Dennison D, Chandy M. Etiology of diarrhea in patients undergoing allogeneic bone marrow transplantation in South India. Transplantation 2002;73:1247–51.
[17] Mori I, Matsumoto K, Sugimoto K, et al. Prolonged shedding of rotavirus in a geriatric inpatient. J Med Virol 2002;67:613–5.
[18] Cunliffe NA, Gondwe JS, Kirkwood CD, et al. Effect of concomitant HIV infection on presentation and outcome of rotavirus gastroenteritis in Malawian children. Lancet 2001; 358:550–5.
[19] Desselberger U. Rotavirus infections: guidelines for treatment and prevention. Drugs 1999; 58:447–52.
[20] Murphy TV, Gargiullo PM, Massoudi MS, et al. Intussusception among infants given an oral rotavirus vaccine. N Engl J Med 2001;344:564–72.
[21] De Vos B, Vesikari T, Linhares AC, et al. A rotavirus vaccine for prophylaxis of infants against rotavirus gastroenteritis. Pediatr Infect Dis J 2004;23(10 Suppl):S179–82.
[22] Clark HF, Bernstein DI, Dennehy PH, et al. Safety, efficacy, and immunogenicity of a live, quadrivalent human-bovine reassortant rotavirus vaccine in healthy infants. J Pediatr 2004; 144:184–90.
[23] Moreno-Espinosa S, Farkas T, Jiang X. Human caliciviruses and pediatric gastroenteritis. Semin Pediatr Infect Dis 2004;15:237–45.

[24] Pang XL, Honma S, Nakata S, Vesikari T. Human caliciviruses in acute gastroenteritis of young children in the community. J Infect Dis 2000;181(Suppl 2):S288–94.
[25] Fankhauser RL, Monroe SS, Noel JS, et al. Epidemiologic and molecular trends of "Norwalk-like viruses" associated with outbreaks of gastroenteritis in the United States. J Infect Dis 2002;186:1–7.
[26] Chadwick PR, McCann R. Transmission of a small round structured virus by vomiting during a hospital outbreak of gastroenteritis. J Hosp Infect 1994;26:251–9.
[27] Chadwick PR, Walker M, Rees AE. Airborne transmission of a small round structured virus. Lancet 1994;343:171.
[28] Atmar RL, Estes MK. Diagnosis of noncultivatable gastroenteritis viruses, the human caliciviruses. Clin Microbiol Rev 2001;14:15–37.
[29] Walter JE, Mitchell DK. Astrovirus infection in children. Curr Opin Infect Dis 2003;16: 247–53.
[30] Glass RI, Noel J, Mitchell D, et al. The changing epidemiology of astrovirus-associated gastroenteritis: a review. Arch Virol 1996;12(Suppl):287–300.
[31] Mitchell DK, Monroe SS, Jiang X, Matson DO, Glass RI, Pickering LK. Virologic features of an astrovirus diarrhea outbreak in a day care center revealed by reverse transcriptase-polymerase chain reaction. J Infect Dis 1995;172:1437–44.
[32] Pinchoff RJ, Kaufman SS, Magid MS, et al. Adenovirus infection in pediatric small bowel transplantation recipients. Transplantation 2003;76:183–9.
[33] Koopman JS, Turkish VJ, Monto AS, Gouvea V, Srivastava S, Isaacson RE. Patterns and etiology of diarrhea in three clinical settings. Am J Epidemiol 1984;119:114–23.
[34] Preliminary FoodNet data on the incidence of infection with pathogens transmitted commonly through food–selected sites, United States, 2003. MMWR Morb Mortal Wkly Rep 2004;53:338–43.
[35] Friedman CR, Hoekstra RM, Samuel M, et al. Risk factors for sporadic *Campylobacter* infection in the United States: a case-control study in FoodNet sites. Clin Infect Dis 2004; 38(Suppl 3):S285–96.
[36] Blaser MJ, Wells JG, Feldman RA, Pollard RA, Allen JR. *Campylobacter* enteritis in the United States: a multicenter study. Ann Intern Med 1983;98:360–5.
[37] Kapperud G, Lassen J, Ostroff SM, Aasen S. Clinical features of sporadic *Campylobacter* infections in Norway. Scand J Infect Dis 1992;24:741–9.
[38] Hellard ME, Sinclair MI, Hogg GG, Fairley CK. Prevalence of enteric pathogens among community based asymptomatic individuals. J Gastroenterol Hepatol 2000;15:290–3.
[39] Guerrant RL, Van Gilder T, Steiner TS, et al. Practice guidelines for the management of infectious diarrhea. Clin Infect Dis 2001;32:331–51.
[40] Daniels NA, MacKinnon L, Rowe SM, Bean NH, Griffin PM, Mead PS. Foodborne disease outbreaks in United States schools. Pediatr Infect Dis J 2002;21:623–8.
[41] Reptile-associated salmonellosis—selected states, 1998–2002. MMWR Morb Mortal Wkly Rep 2003;52:1206–9.
[42] Broide E, Shapiro M, Boldur I, et al. Salmonellosis: an epidemiologic study. Isr Med Assoc J 2005;7:91–4.
[43] Levine OS, Levine MM. Houseflies (*Musca domestica*) as mechanical vectors of shigellosis. Rev Infect Dis 1991;13:688–96.
[44] Rowe PC, Orrbine E, Lior H, et al. Risk of hemolytic uremic syndrome after sporadic *Escherichia coli* O157:H7 infection: Results of a Canadian collaborative study. Investigators of the Canadian Pediatric Kidney Disease Research Center. J Pediatr 1998; 132:777–82.
[45] Tarr PI, Gordon CA, Chandler WL. Shiga-toxin-producing *Escherichia coli* and haemolytic uraemic syndrome. Lancet 2005;365:1073–86.
[46] Safdar N, Said A, Gangnon RE, Maki DG. Risk of hemolytic uremic syndrome after antibiotic treatment of *Escherichia coli* O157:H7 enteritis: a meta-analysis. JAMA 2002;288: 996–1001.

[47] Drugs for parasitic infections. New Rochelle (NY): The Medical Letter; 2004.
[48] Chappell CL, Okhuysen PC. Cryptosporidiosis. Curr Opin Infect Dis 2002;15:523–7.
[49] Smith HV, Corcoran GD. New drugs and treatment for cryptosporidiosis. Curr Opin Infect Dis 2004;17:557–64.
[50] Practice parameter: the management of acute gastroenteritis in young children. American Academy of Pediatrics, Provisional Committee on Quality Improvement, Subcommittee on Acute Gastroenteritis. Pediatrics 1996;97:424–35.
[51] Subbotina MD, Timchenko VN, Vorobyov MM, Konunova YS, Aleksandrovih YS, Shushunov S. Effect of oral administration of tormentil root extract (*Potentilla tormentilla*) on rotavirus diarrhea in children: a randomized, double blind, controlled trial. Pediatr Infect Dis J 2003;22:706–11.
[52] Sullivan A, Nord CE. Probiotics and gastrointestinal diseases. J Intern Med 2005;257:78–92.
[53] The Jordan report 20th anniversary accelerated development of vaccines. Bethesda (MD): US Department of Health and Human Services, National Institutes of Health; 2002.

ELSEVIER
SAUNDERS

Infect Dis Clin N Am 19 (2005) 603–615

INFECTIOUS
DISEASE CLINICS
OF NORTH AMERICA

Neonatal Candidiasis

P. Brian Smith, MD[a,b], William J. Steinbach, MD[a], Daniel K. Benjamin, Jr, MD, MPH, PhD[a,b,*]

[a]*Department of Pediatrics, Duke University Medical Center, Durham, NC 27710, USA*

[b]*Duke Clinical Research Institute, Duke University Medical Center, Durham, NC 27710, USA*

Epidemiology

Documented invasive candidiasis is defined as a positive culture from normally sterile body fluid. The most common source (approximately 70% of neonatal cases) is the bloodstream. Other common sources include urine obtained by catheterization or suprapubic aspiration (15%) and cerebrospinal fluid (approximately 10%). Other fluids, including peritoneal fluid, are uncommon sources and account for approximately 5% of cases.

The cumulative incidence of invasive candidiasis is inversely proportional to birth weight (eg, neonates born > 1500 g, < 1%; neonates born 1001–1500 g, 1%; neonates born 751–1000 g, 4%; and neonates born 401–750 g, 12%). These incidences have been consistent from reports of the Neonatal Research Network [1,2] and the Pediatrix group [3]. Nearly 80% of cases diagnosed in premature infants occur in the first 42 days of life [2]. Birth weight and age at time of infection also predict subsequent mortality; 40% of neonates weighing less than 750 g die compared with less than 20% in neonates weighing 1000 to 1500 g. The associated mortality with invasive candidiasis is three times higher than that of uninfected infants of similar gestational age and birth weight [4]. In addition to postconceptual age, species of infecting organism (*Pseudomonas* > *Candida albicans* > enteric gram-negative rods > *Candida parapsilosis* > gram-positive cocci) is the strongest predictor of subsequent mortality in

Dr. Smith received support from the National Institutes of Health T32 (AI 052080). Dr. Steinbach received support from the National Institute of Allergy and Infectious Diseases 1 K08 (A1061149-01). Dr. Benjamin received support from the National Institute of Child Health and Human Development (HD044799).

* Corresponding author. PO Box 17969, Duke Clinical Research Institute, Durham, NC 27715, USA

E-mail address: danny.benjamin@duke.edu (D.K. Benjamin).

doi:10.1016/j.idc.2005.05.007

id.theclinics.com

neonatal nosocomial bloodstream infections. Morbidity associated with invasive candidiasis also is substantial, with end-organ damage [5] and neurodevelopmental impairment common [2,6].

Candida colonization can be detected in approximately 30% of infants weighing less than 1500 g birth weight. Similar to invasive disease, colonization increases with decreasing birth weight and gestational age [7]. Several studies have found colonization to be a risk factor, but have not always identified it before infection. In the largest prospective multicenter study of colonization, colonization was *not* an independent risk factor for subsequent candidiasis [8]. Colonization acquisition occurs over time in the nursery, and many infants who are not colonized in the first days of life acquire colonization during their stay.

Risk factors for invasive disease [8] have been described, but ascertainment of many of these risk factors may not have clinical application to guide systematic prophylaxis. The highest risk period for candidiasis in a premature infant is 3 through 42 days of life. Risk factors are likely to be crucial to the pathophysiology of development of disease, but early in this high-risk period these factors either often are unknown (eg, colonization) or are commonly present (eg, central vascular access), and so reliance on the presence of these risk factors to guide prophylaxis may not be helpful.

Prophylaxis

Prophylaxis with oral antifungal agents in premature infants has had limited success. These limitations have been in the application, safety, and side effects in infants weighing less than 1000 g [9–11]. Because of lack of success with oral agents, use of systemic antifungal agents has been pursued.

The pharmacokinetics of fluconazole makes it an excellent drug for prophylaxis. It has a long half-life, high cerebrospinal fluid penetration, low protein binding, and saliva and lung levels are 1.3 and 1.2 times that of plasma levels, providing higher levels at key areas of colonization [12,13]. The pharmacokinetics of fluconazole theoretically allow for long dosing intervals, excellent tissue penetration, and easy elimination. Antifungal pharmacokinetic data in premature infants, especially in neonates born weighing less than 750 g, are extremely limited. Saxen et al [14] studied preterm infants (birth weight range 750–1100 g) and reported fluconazole plasma half-lives in the first 2 weeks of life (88.6 hours), at 2 weeks of life (55 hours), and thereafter (21.4 hours). The safety of fluconazole is well documented in older patients, and the product is thought to be safe in neonates. Systematic studies in premature infants have been limited, and most have been single center with 100 infants or less.

Emergence of fluconazole resistance and diversification of *Candida* species are major concerns in prophylaxis strategies. The development of fluconazole resistance in older patients exposed to prophylaxis has been mixed [15,16]. Kicklighter et al [17] evaluated resistance to fluconazole in neonates in their prophylaxis study and reported that isolates of *C albicans* remained sensitive to fluconazole with mean minimal inhibitory concentration values less than 2 μg/mL.

Fluconazole prophylaxis can lead to the emergence of *Candida* species other than *C albicans* and *C parapsilosis*—the leading causes of candidiasis in the nursery, both of which are largely susceptible to fluconazole. Species diversification is an important concern because mortality varies so substantially by species. Diversification has occurred in older patients exposed to prophylaxis, resulting in more frequent isolation of *Candida glabrata,* an organism with a high mortality rate. Some diversification of species as a result of fluconazole prophylaxis (eg, resistance) seems inevitable and requires careful study. Resistance, diversification, and subsequent mortality are key questions that must be addressed before widespread implementation of a potentially useful practice.

The efficacy of fluconazole in the nursery is promising but unproven; pilot data indicate that the product requires definitive evaluation. In a randomized study of 103 preterm very-low-birth-weight (VLBW, < 1500 g) infants, intravenous fluconazole decreased rectal colonization, but did not decrease the incidence of invasive candidiasis [17]. Kaufman et al [18] randomized 100 neonates less than 1000 g birth weight (with either central vascular access or endotracheal tube) in a single-center study. Fluconazole colonization was monitored via weekly surveillance, and antifungal susceptibility testing results of the *Candida* isolates did not change during the study. Invasive candidiasis occurred in 20% (10 of 50) of the infants in the placebo group and none (0 of 50) of the infants in the fluconazole group. After the 6-week treatment period, invasive candidiasis occurred in three infants in the placebo group and one in the fluconazole group.

The placebo arm in this single-center study had one of the highest incidence rates (13 of 50 [26%]) of invasive candidiasis reported in neonates less than 1000 g birth weight. A cumulative incidence of 26% in neonates less than 1000 g birth weight is higher than any of the 16 centers of the Neonatal Research Network (even limited to infants with a central catheter or endotracheal tube in place) and is higher than any of the 100 centers in the Pediatrix collaborative studies [2,3].

The prophylaxis studies mentioned in detail previously [17,18] were well designed, but several important aspects of design were not incorporated, as follows:

1. Neither study collected pharmacokinetic data.
2. Both studies were completed at one center. Single-center studies conducted in neonatology should be interpreted with caution given the wide variability in neonatal care and outcomes among nurseries [19].
3. Neither study included death as a part of the primary end point. Death should be included with the development of candidiasis as a part of the

composite end point because death is a competing end point—an infant who dies at 10 days of life cannot develop candidiasis at 12 days of life.

4. Both studies included relatively low-risk patients; the incidence of candidiasis in neonates weighing 750 to 1500 g is 1% to 4%.
5. Both studies had incidences of invasive candidiasis inconsistent with the median incidence reported from large multicenter collaborative efforts.
6. Neither study provided neurodevelopmental follow-up.
7. Neither study provided multicenter data regarding resistance and species diversification The crucial questions yet to be answered regarding fluconazole prophylaxis in neonates reflect basic tenets of drug development, and each deserves an answer:
   1. What is the minimum effective dose of fluconazole?
   2. Is 6 weeks of prophylaxis safe in this patient population?
   3. Does prophylaxis work, and what is the ideal patient population (eg, <750 g, <1000 g, use of risk factors)?
   4. Does prophylaxis cause resistance whereby more infants eventually have incurable invasive candidiasis?

Given the prior pilot data and substantial data generated from epidemiologic cohort studies, some of which have 18 to 22 month neurodevelopment follow-up, a multicenter pivotal study is necessary. This study should include pharmacokinetic evaluation to determine the minimum effective dose. It also should include 18 to 22 months' neurodevelopmental follow-up and should assess antifungal resistance, *Candida* species diversification, and resistance-related morbidity and mortality.

Treatment

There is a paucity of randomized trials evaluating treatment options in neonatal candidiasis, and a well-powered efficacy trial has not been completed. As in older patients, removal of a central venous catheter within 24 hours of a positive blood culture is an important component of treatment [20]. Delayed removal of central venous catheters in candidemic neonates has been associated with increased mortality and morbidity, including worse neurodevelopmental outcomes [20–22]. One analysis of Neonatal Research Network data reported significantly increased rates of death and neurodevelopmental impairment in infants whose catheters were removed after more than 1 day of antifungal therapy [21].

Amphotericin B deoxycholate

A polyene antifungal, amphotericin B, has been the antifungal standard of care for nearly 50 years. The antifungal is often used for empirical therapy and is the most often used first-line agent for invasive candidiasis in neonates [23]. Despite amphotericin B's place as the "gold standard," there are limited pharmacokinetic data in neonates and some noticeable differences in adult versus pediatric patients. Two studies involving a total of 17 neonates showed longer half-life of the drug than the half-life observed in adults [24,25]. The dose of amphotericin B is 0.5 to 1 mg/kg once daily over 2 to 4 hours [26]. Test doses are not required because the drug is better tolerated in neonates than in adults [27]. Cerebrospinal fluid penetration, which is only 5% to 10% of serum levels in adults, reaches 40% to 90% of serum levels in preterm neonates [24]. Side effects observed in neonates include electrolyte abnormalities and nephrotoxicity [28]. Close monitoring of potassium, magnesium, and renal function is important during therapy [29]. Amphotericin B is effective against most *Candida* species causing disease in neonates except for *C lusitaniae* [30], and resistance has been noted in some isolates of *C glabrata* and *C krusei* [31]. A prospective observational study of 59 infants with invasive candidiasis found that all isolates were sensitive to amphotericin B [32].

Lipid preparations of amphotericin B

Inability to tolerate amphotericin B deoxycholate because of renal insufficiency may provoke the need for alternate therapies for invasive candidiasis [33]. Three lipid formulations of amphotericin B are available: amphotericin B lipid complex (ABLC or Abelcet), amphotericin B colloidal dispersion (ABCD or Amphotec), and liposomal amphotericin B (L-amB or AmBisome). An advantage of these drugs is the ability to administer increased doses of the parent drug amphotericin B with less associated renal toxicity. This decrease in toxicity may be due to the release of the drug by lipases elaborated by inflammatory cells at the infection site [34]. Published experience with these drugs in neonates is limited [27]. There is some concern about the ability of the lipid preparations to clear renal infections because the drugs concentrate in lesser amounts in the kidney than does amphotericin B deoxycholate [35,36].

In the only randomized trial involving these antifungals in neonates, ABCD and L-amB were compared with amphotericin B deoxycholate in 56 candidemic infants, including 36 VLBW infants (birth weight <1000 g) [33]. Infants with creatinine less than 1.2 mg/dL were given amphotericin B deoxycholate ($n = 34$), whereas the remaining patients were randomized to either ABCD ($n = 16$) or L-AmB ($n = 6$). No differences in mortality or time to clear infection were observed, and no side effects were noted in either group of infants.

In another study, L-amB was evaluated in 40 preterm and 4 term infants with candidiasis [29]. The only side effect noted was hypokalemia, which occurred in 16 (36%) of the neonates. All of the neonates responded to potassium supplementation. Successful therapy was observed in 32 (73%) of the infants, including 5 of 6 (83%) infants with meningitis. All the infants who died were in the preterm group. Another series of 41 episodes of candidiasis in neonates (69% were VLBW), identified and treated prospectively with L-amB, noted successful treatment in 39 cases [27]. One infant died as a result of candidal sepsis, and a second infant died as a result of *Klebsiella*. Another infant required the addition of fluconazole to clear the infection. Transient liver function abnormalities were noted in only one patient, and no infant was removed from therapy because of side effects. The authors noted that eradication of infection occurred earlier when the target dose of 5 to 7 mg/kg/day was reached faster and concluded that clinicians should initiate therapy with this dose.

ABLC given to 11 infants intolerant of or failing treatment with amphotericin B deoxycholate resulted in a mortality rate of 18% (2 of 11) [37]. One of the infants died of candidiasis, but the other neonate had cleared the infection before death. No side effects of the drug were noted. In a multicenter pediatric trial of 111 patients on ABLC, the only side effect noted in the 11 neonates was a mild increase in serum creatinine in 36% (4 of 11) of the patients [38]. Another trial observed 118 cases of neonatal candidiasis in which L-amB was given to 8 neonates, and ABLC was given to 29 neonates [39]. No difference in mortality was observed between the two groups, and efficacy was 94% and 86% with L-amB and ABLC.

Flucytosine

Flucytosine is not recommended as monotherapy because resistance develops rapidly, but the antifungal is given occasionally in combination with amphotericin B for central nervous system infections [40]. Although there are no pediatric studies focusing on flucytosine, a review of 17 cases of candidal meningitis (including 11 patients <12 months old) observed improvement in 15 patients on combination therapy of amphotericin B and flucytosine [41]. In Neonatal Research Network data that evaluated 320 VLBW infants with candidiasis [21], including 27 of 320 with meningitis, time to clear infection was longer in infants given combination flucytosine and amphotericin B than in infants treated with amphotericin B alone. Because the sample size was small and neither cerebrospinal fluid evaluation nor therapy was standardized, the authors advised caution in interpreting this finding.

The lack of a parenteral formulation limits the utility of flucytosine. The drug is dosed at 50 to 150 mg/kg/day divided every 6 hours. Bone marrow suppression is the predominant toxicity, seen largely with levels greater than 100 μg/mL, so levels should be monitored closely in patients with impaired renal function [42,43]. Transient elevation in liver function tests also has been seen in adult patients. We have observed episodes of necrotizing enterocolitis in neonates on flucytosine therapy. The drug should be used with extreme caution in preterm neonates because the benefits are unproven, and the risks associated with therapy are not trivial.

Fluconazole and voriconazole

Fluconazole, a triazole member of the azole antifungal family, also is commonly used to treat candidiasis in infants [44]. The drug may be given orally or parenterally and is nearly completely absorbed from the gastrointestinal tract [17,44]. The drug has a long half-life that decreases with increasing postnatal age [14]. Although fungistatic, fluconazole penetrates the cerebrospinal fluid, kidneys, and liver well. Fluconazole is ideal for treating urinary tract infections because it is concentrated and excreted predominantly unchanged by the kidneys.

Fluconazole compared favorably with amphotericin B deoxycholate in one small randomized trial of VLBW infants [45]. Although the study was insufficiently powered for noninferiority, there was no observed difference in survival between the two groups. Elevated transaminases were observed in the amphotericin B group, and the fluconazole group used central venous catheters for shorter periods, presumably because of the availability of the oral formulation.

Other reports of fluconazole use are from uncontrolled prospective studies or retrospective reports. In one study that included 32 patients younger than 3 months of age with reported outcomes, 31 experienced successful treatment with fluconazole [46]. Two of the patients had elevated transaminases during treatment. Another group of 19 preterm infants treated with fluconazole experienced clearance of infection in 18 cases (95%) [47].

The recommended dosage of the intravenous or oral form of the drug in adult patients is approximately 4.5 to 6 mg/kg/day, but dosages of 10 to 12 mg/kg/day have been used for treatment in pediatric and neonatal patients. Although it is important to monitor for severe hepatotoxicity, generally only mild elevations of transaminases are seen. The two most common species of *Candida* found in neonates, *C albicans* and *C parapsilosis,* are usually sensitive to fluconazole. Fifty percent of *C glabrata* and 100% of *C krusei* isolates have been reported to be resistant to fluconazole, however [48].

Voriconazole is a second-generation triazole, a derivative of fluconazole, and is available in intravenous and oral forms. The drug has a broader spectrum of antifungal activity against *Candida* species than fluconazole. Voriconazole has been found to be active in vitro against *C glabrata* and *C krusei* and some isolates that have developed resistance to fluconazole. Voriconazole should be used with caution, however, in instances in which fluconazole resistance is likely [49]. To emphasize this point, we have observed one infant at our institution that developed resistance to both azoles while on treatment doses of fluconazole. Voriconazole is not recommended in patients with renal insufficiency because its cyclodextrin carrier is cleared renally [50]. The drug is metabolized by the liver, and good cerebrospinal fluid penetration has been observed. Torsades de pointes has been seen rarely during therapy in adult patients. Other side effects include allergic reactions, elevated transaminases, and visual disturbances.

Voriconazole has not been studied in infants. In a preterm neonate with a developing retina and at risk for retinopathy of prematurity, the visual disturbances are especially concerning [51]. Because the pharmacokinetics and safety in neonates are unknown for this product, we have used it only in the face of documented resistance or extreme clinical circumstances.

Echinocandins: caspofungin, micafungin, and anidulafungin

The echinocandins interfere with cell wall integrity as an inhibitor of 1,3-β-D-glucan synthase [52]. This drug class is available only in the intravenous preparation and is fungicidal for all medically important *Candida* species in neonates, with the possible exception of *C parapsilosis,* for which it may be fungistatic [53]. The first of these to be licensed, caspofungin, was not tested in neonates before market approval. To date, there remains very little experience with the drug in the neonatal population. Odio et al [52] reported a series of 10 neonates (9 preterm) in whom caspofungin was used as salvage therapy after initial therapy with amphotericin B deoxycholate. In that report, 9 of 10 (90%) infants survived, and no adverse drug events were observed. One patient experienced a relapse 4 days after the last dose of caspofungin, but subsequently cleared the infection with a second course of therapy with caspofungin. The infants were given a dose of 1 mg/kg/day for 2 days, then 2 mg/kg/day for the duration of treatment; 80% of the isolates in the study were resistant to fluconazole.

Although no pharmacokinetic data were obtained in this study, increased clearance of the drug has been observed in pediatric patients relative to adults [54]. In this series of patients (age 2–17 years), weight-based dosing using 1 mg/kg/day yielded suboptimal levels. The data suggested that a body surface area approach using daily maintenance doses of 50 mg/m^2/day was necessary to obtain appropriate drug levels.

Side effects of caspofungin seem to be minimal because the target enzyme, 1,3-β-D-glucan synthase, is not present in humans [55]. In a trial of caspofungin versus amphotericin B deoxycholate for candidiasis in adult patients, only 3% of patients on caspofungin therapy withdrew from the study because of side effects compared with 23% of patients receiving amphotericin B [56]. A retrospective review of 25 pediatric patients receiving the drug found caspofungin to be well tolerated in this population [57]. Only three patients experienced side effects possibly related to caspofungin, including hypokalemia, anemia, and elevated liver function tests.

Micafungin is likely to be the second echinocandin to gain US Food and Drug Administration approval. The pharmacokinetics have been described in older children and in premature infants. Older children received 4 mg/kg/day, and serial blood samples were collected on day 1 and day 4 [58]. The area under the plasma concentration-time curves (AUC) was dose proportional in older children (at least in children >4 years old). AUC increased proportionally with dose, and half-life (11–17 hours) did not vary with time.

Micafungin was evaluated in premature infants in a single-dose pharmacokinetic study completed within the National Institute of Child Health and Human Development–sponsored Pediatric Pharmacology Research Network [59]. The half-life was 8 hours in neonates weighing greater than 1000 g and 5.5 hours in neonates weighing 500 to 1000 g. The AUC in neonates weighing greater than 1000 g was approximately 50% less than that observed in older children; the AUC was approximately 50% less in neonates weighing 500 to 1000 g compared with neonates weighing greater than 1000 g. The substantially reduced AUC observed in neonates is extremely important because the echinocandins (as a class) have shown a dose-response relationship. As of this writing, the appropriate dosage of any of the echinocandins in neonates is not known, and the kinetics of micafungin suggests that infants may need larger than expected dosages.

Anidulafungin is the third echinocandin in late-phase testing; adult dosages under study are 50 mg/day for esophageal candidiasis and 100 mg/day for invasive candidiasis. The product has been studied in children age 2 to 17 and the pharmacokinetics described [60]. Children received 0.75 or 1.5 mg/kg/day (2 $\times$ loading dose), and blood was taken after the first and fifth dose. Anidulafungin (similar to micafungin) was observed to be safe and well tolerated. Weight-adjusted clearance, concentrations, and AUC were consistent across age. Steady-state concentrations were reached after the first dose. The product has yet to be evaluated in neonates.

Echinocandins and neonatal meningoencephalitis

Meningoencephalitis is a common component of neonatal candidiasis, and the echinocandins are likely to have minimal penetration into the cerebrospinal fluid of neonates. Several cases of the successful use of echinocandins in central nervous system infections have been published, however. Also, there are animal model data on the efficacy of echinocandins in central nervous system infections.

Similar to amphotericin B deoxycholate, micafungin was not detectable in the cerebrospinal fluid in neutropenic rabbit models [61]. Both products have lower levels in the brain than in other tissue sites. Therapeutic drug levels of amphotericin B and micafungin have been documented, however, in central nervous system infections in neutropenic rabbits as documented by successful treatment [62]. Echinocandins (similar to amphotericin B) are not detectable at high levels in the cerebrospinal fluid, but they do penetrate the brain tissue at normally observed plasma concentrations and dosages that reflect the adult dosages used to treat invasive candidiasis. The echinocandins are able to treat animal model central nervous system infections successfully.

The data from the same animal modeling system for amphotericin B deoxycholate and L-AmB [63] predicted closely the clearance of *Candida* in human patients with *Candida* meningoencephalitis. These animal studies provide proof of principle that amphotericin B deoxycholate can be used successfully in the treatment of central nervous system infections in humans. Likewise, animal model data of the echinocandins may predict clinical response in adults and infants.

This proof of principle has been observed clinically with the echinocandins in a case series of 10 neonates with refractory candidemia despite antifungal therapy [52]. One neonate had right-sided endocarditis, one had renal involvement, and one had meningitis. The echinocandin cleared the infection in all cases, including prompt resolution of the positive CSF cultures.

Although the data on the echinocandins for the treatment of neonatal meningitis are limited, the information on amphotericin B and fluconazole for the treatment of neonatal meningitis is limited as well. Most of the data for the antifungal treatment of neonatal candidiasis also are limited to animal models, clinical case reports, and the occasional case series. Even in these reports, reliable time to clearance and mycologic efficacy for any antifungal (amphotericin B, the echinocandins, or fluconazole) are not available to practicing neonatologists. These reports primarily consist of case series reporting X_1 treated neonates, and of these, X_2 survived.

It remains to be seen what the optimal therapy for neonatal meningoencephalitis should be, and if the echinocandins will be as successful in the treatment of neonatal candidiasis as they have been in the treatment of older patients. The echinocandins are an exciting class of products for the treatment of candidiasis and have been safe and effective in older patients. The pharmacokinetics, safety, and efficacy in neonates are unknown, however. If the clinician elects to use one of the products, consultation with pharmacokinetics expertise is warranted until further dosing and safety data are published.

Summary

For prophylaxis and treatment of neonatal candidiasis, fundamental questions remain regarding dosing, safety, and efficacy. These questions require multicenter collaborative efforts and basic knowledge in pharmacology, pathophysiology, and epidemiology. Prior research efforts have provided the field with much of the basic knowledge to move forward in multicenter collaborative research. It is now incumbent on clinicians, clinical researchers, industry, and government agencies to collaborate to answer the clinical questions vital to the prevention and treatment of neonatal candidiasis.

References

[1] Stoll BJ, Hansen N, Fanaroff AA, et al. Late-onset sepsis in very low birth weight neonates: the experience of the NICHD Neonatal Research Network. Pediatrics 2002;110(2 Pt 1): 285–91.

[2] Benjamin DK Jr, Stoll BJ, Fanaroff AA, et al. Neonatal candidiasis among extremely low birth weight infants: risk factors, mortality, and neuro-developmental outcomes at 18–22 months. Pediatrics 2005; accepted for publication.

[3] Benjamin DK Jr, DeLong ER, Steinbach WJ, Cotton CM, Walsh TJ, Clark RH. Empirical therapy for neonatal candidemia in very low birth weight infants. Pediatrics 2003;112(3 Pt 1): 543–7.
[4] Benjamin DK, DeLong E, Cotten CM, Garges HP, Steinbach WJ, Clark RH. Mortality following blood culture in premature infants: increased with gram-negative bacteremia and candidemia, but not gram-positive bacteremia. J Perinatol 2004;24:175–80.
[5] Benjamin DK Jr, Poole C, Steinbach WJ, Rowen JL, Walsh TJ. Neonatal candidemia and end-organ damage: a critical appraisal of the literature using meta-analytic techniques. Pediatrics 2003;112(3 Pt 1):634–40.
[6] Friedman S, Richardson SE, Jacobs SE, O'Brien K. Systemic *Candida* infection in extremely low birth weight infants: short term morbidity and long term neurodevelopmental outcome. Pediatr Infect Dis J 2000;19:499–504.
[7] Saiman L, Ludington E, Dawson JD, et al. Risk factors for *Candida* species colonization of neonatal intensive care unit patients. Pediatr Infect Dis J 2001;20:1119–24.
[8] Saiman L, Ludington E, Pfaller M, et al. Risk factors for candidemia in neonatal intensive care unit patients. The National Epidemiology of Mycosis Survey study group. Pediatr Infect Dis J 2000;19:319–24.
[9] Damjanovic V, Connolly CM, van Saene HK, et al. Selective decontamination with nystatin for control of a *Candida* outbreak in a neonatal intensive care unit. J Hosp Infect 1993;24: 245–59.
[10] Sims ME, Yoo Y, You H, Salminen C, Walther FJ. Prophylactic oral nystatin and fungal infections in very-low-birthweight infants. Am J Perinatol 1988;5:33–6.
[11] Wainer S, Cooper PA, Funk E, Bental RY, Sandler DA, Patel J. Prophylactic miconazole oral gel for the prevention of neonatal fungal rectal colonization and systemic infection. Pediatr Infect Dis J 1992;11:713–6.
[12] Koks CH, Crommentuyn KM, Hoetelmans RM, Mathot RA, Beijnen JH. Can fluconazole concentrations in saliva be used for therapeutic drug monitoring? Ther Drug Monit 2001;23: 449–53.
[13] Vaden SL, Heit MC, Hawkins EC, Manaugh C, Riviere JE. Fluconazole in cats: pharmacokinetics following intravenous and oral administration and penetration into cerebrospinal fluid, aqueous humour and pulmonary epithelial lining fluid. J Vet Pharmacol Ther 1997;20:181–6.
[14] Saxen H, Hoppu K, Pohjavuori M. Pharmacokinetics of fluconazole in very low birth weight infants during the first two weeks of life. Clin Pharmacol Therap 1993;54:269–77.
[15] Rex JH, Rinaldi MG, Pfaller MA. Resistance of *Candida* species to fluconazole. Antimicrob Agents Chemother 1995;39:1–8.
[16] Lewis RE, Klepser ME. The changing face of nosocomial candidemia: epidemiology, resistance, and drug therapy. Am J Health Syst Pharm 1999;56:525–33.
[17] Kicklighter SD, Springer SC, Cox T, Hulsey TC, Turner RB. Fluconazole for prophylaxis against candidal rectal colonization in the very low birth weight infant. Pediatrics 2001;107: 293–8.
[18] Kaufman D, Boyle R, Hazen KC, Patrie JT, Robinson M, Donowitz LG. Fluconazole prophylaxis against fungal colonization and infection in preterm infants. N Engl J Med 2001; 345:1660–6.
[19] Walsh-Sukys MC, Tyson JE, Wright LL, et al. Persistent pulmonary hypertension of the newborn in the era before nitric oxide: practice variation and outcomes. Pediatrics 2000; 105(1 Pt 1):14–20.
[20] Eppes SC, Troutman JL, Gutman LT. Outcome of treatment of candidemia in children whose central catheters were removed or retained. Pediatr Infect Dis J 1989;8:99–104.
[21] Benjamin DK Jr, Stoll BJ, Fanaroff AA, et al. Neonatal candidiasis among infants $<$ 1000 g birthweight: risk factors, mortality, and neuro-developmental outcomes at 18–22 months. Presented at Interscience Conference on Antimicrobial Agents and Chemotherapy. Washington, DC, 2004.

[22] Karlowicz MG, Rowen JL, Barnes-Eley ML, et al. The role of birth weight and gestational age in distinguishing extremely low birth weight infants at high risk of developing candidemia from infants at low risk: a multicenter study [abstract]. Pediatr Res 2002;51:301A.
[23] Rowen JL, Tate JM. Management of neonatal candidiasis. Neonatal Candidiasis Study Group. Pediatr Infect Dis J 1998;17:1007–11.
[24] Baley JE, Meyers C, Kliegman RM, Jacobs MR, Blumer JL. Pharmacokinetics, outcome of treatment, and toxic effects of amphotericin B and 5-fluorocytosine in neonates. J Pediatr 1990;116:791–7.
[25] Starke JR, Mason EO Jr, Kramer WG, Kaplan SL. Pharmacokinetics of amphotericin B in infants and children. J Infect Dis 1987;155:766–74.
[26] Serra G, Mezzano P, Bonacci W. Therapeutic treatment of systemic candidiasis in newborns. J Chemother 1991;3(Suppl 1):240–4.
[27] Juster-Reicher A, Flidel-Rimon O, Amitay M, Even-Tov S, Shinwell E, Leibovitz E. High-dose liposomal amphotericin B in the therapy of systemic candidiasis in neonates. Eur J Clin Microbiol Infect Dis 2003;22:603–7.
[28] Baley JE, Kliegman RM, Fanaroff AA. Disseminated fungal infections in very low-birth-weight infants: therapeutic toxicity. Pediatrics 1984;73:153–7.
[29] Scarcella A, Pasquariello MB, Giugliano B, Vendemmia M, de Lucia A. Liposomal amphotericin B treatment for neonatal fungal infections. Pediatr Infect Dis J 1998;17:146–8.
[30] Minari A, Hachem R, Raad I. *Candida lusitaniae*: a cause of breakthrough fungemia in cancer patients. Clin Infect Dis 2001;32:186–90.
[31] Pfaller MA, Diekema DJ, Jones RN, Messer SA, Hollis RJ. Trends in antifungal susceptibility of *Candida* spp. isolated from pediatric and adult patients with bloodstream infections: SENTRY Antimicrobial Surveillance Program, 1997 to 2000. J Clin Microbiol 2002;40:852–6.
[32] Roilides E, Farmaki E, Evdoridou J, et al. Neonatal candidiasis: analysis of epidemiology, drug susceptibility, and molecular typing of causative isolates. Eur J Clin Microbiol Infect Dis 2004;23:745–50.
[33] Linder N, Klinger G, Shalit I, et al. Treatment of candidaemia in premature infants: comparison of three amphotericin B preparations. J Antimicrob Chemother 2003;52:663–7.
[34] Swenson CE, Perkins WR, Roberts P, et al. In vitro and in vivo antifungal activity of amphotericin B lipid complex: are phospholipases important? Antimicrob Agents Chemother 1998;42:767–71.
[35] Bekersky I, Fielding RM, Dressler DE, Lee JW, Buell DN, Walsh TJ. Pharmacokinetics, excretion, and mass balance of liposomal amphotericin B (AmBisome) and amphotericin B deoxycholate in humans. Antimicrob Agents Chemother 2002;46:828–33.
[36] Biyikli NK, Tugtepe H, Akpmar I, Alpay H, Ozek E. The longest use of liposomal amphotericin B and 5-fluorocytosine. Pediatr Nephrol 2004;19:801–4.
[37] Adler-Shohet F, Waskin H, Lieberman JM. Amphotericin B lipid complex for neonatal invasive candidiasis. Arch Dis Child Fetal Neonatal Ed 2001;84:F131–3.
[38] Walsh TJ, Seibel NL, Arndt C, et al. Amphotericin B lipid complex in pediatric patients with invasive fungal infections. Pediatr Infect Dis J 1999;18:702–8.
[39] Lopez Sastre JB, Coto Cotallo GD, Fernandez Colomer B. Neonatal invasive candidiasis: a prospective multicenter study of 118 cases. Am J Perinatol 2003;20:153–63.
[40] Rao HK, Myers GJ. *Candida* meningitis in the newborn. South Med J 1979;72:1468–71.
[41] Smego RA Jr, Perfect JR, Durack DT. Combined therapy with amphotericin B and 5-fluorocytosine for *Candida* meningitis. Rev Infect Dis 1984;6:791–801.
[42] Frattarelli DA, Reed MD, Giacoia GP, Aranda JV. Antifungals in systemic neonatal candidiasis. Drugs 2004;64:949–68.
[43] Anderson DC, Pickering LK, Feigin RD. Leukocyte function in normal and infected neonates. J Pediatr 1974;85:420–5.
[44] Wenzl TG, Schefels J, Hornchen H, Skopnik H. Pharmacokinetics of oral fluconazole in premature infants. Eur J Pediatr 1998;157:661–2.

[45] Driessen M, Ellis JB, Cooper PA, et al. Fluconazole vs. amphotericin B for the treatment of neonatal fungal septicemia: a prospective randomized trial. Pediatr Infect Dis J 1996;15: 1107–12.
[46] Fasano C, O'Keeffe J, Gibbs D. Fluconazole treatment of neonates and infants with severe fungal infections not treatable with conventional agents. Eur J Clin Microbiol Infect Dis 1994;13:351–4.
[47] Wainer S, Cooper PA, Gouws H, Akierman A. Prospective study of fluconazole therapy in systemic neonatal fungal infection. Pediatr Infect Dis J 1997;16:763–7.
[48] Rowen JL, Tate JM, Nordoff N, Passarell L, McGinnis MR. *Candida* isolates from neonates: frequency of misidentification and reduced fluconazole susceptibility. J Clin Microbiol 1999; 37:3735–7.
[49] Muller FM, Weig M, Peter J, Walsh TJ. Azole cross-resistance to ketoconazole, fluconazole, itraconazole and voriconazole in clinical *Candida albicans* isolates from HIV-infected children with oropharyngeal candidosis. J Antimicrob Chemother 2000;46:338–40.
[50] Sabo JA, Abdel-Rahman SM. Voriconazole: a new triazole antifungal. Ann Pharmacother 2000;34:1032–43.
[51] Groll AH, Gea-Banacloche JC, Glasmacher A, Just-Nuebling G, Maschmeyer G, Walsh TJ. Clinical pharmacology of antifungal compounds. Infect Dis Clin North Am 2003;17:159–91.
[52] Odio CM, Araya R, Pinto LE, et al. Caspofungin therapy of neonates with invasive candidiasis. Pediatr Infect Dis J 2004;23:1093–7.
[53] Vazquez JA, Lynch M, Boikov D, Sobel JD. In vitro activity of a new pneumocandin antifungal, L-743,872, against azole-susceptible and -resistant *Candida* species. Antimicrob Agents Chemother 1997;41:1612–4.
[54] Walsh TJ, Adamson PC, Seibel NL, et al, Pharmacokinetics of caspofungin in pediatric patients [abstract]. Presented at Interscience Conference on Antimicrobial Agents and Chemotherapy. San Diego, CA, 2002.
[55] Walsh TJ, Viviani MA, Arathoon E, et al. New targets and delivery systems for antifungal therapy. Med Mycol 2000;38(Suppl 1):335–47.
[56] Mora-Duarte J, Betts R, Rotstein C, et al. Comparison of caspofungin and amphotericin B for invasive candidiasis. N Engl J Med 2002;347:2020–9.
[57] Franklin JA, McCormick J, Flynn PM. Retrospective study of the safety of caspofungin in immunocompromised pediatric patients. Pediatr Infect Dis J 2003;22:747–9.
[58] Towsend R, Bekersky I, Buell D, Seibel N. Pharmacokinetic (PK) evaluation of echinocandin FK463 in pediatric and adult patients. Presented at Focus on Fungal Infections. Washington (DC), 2001.
[59] Heresi G, Gerstmann D, Blumer J, et al. A pharmacokinetic study of micafungin (FK463) in premature infants [abstract]. Presented at Pediatric Academic Society. Seattle, 2003.
[60] Benjamin DK, Driscoll T, Siebel N, et al, Safety and pharmacokinetics of anidulafungin in pediatric patients with neutropenia. Presented at Interscience Conference on Antimicrobial Agents and Chemotherapy. Washington (DC), 2004.
[61] Groll AH, Mickiene D, Petraitis V, et al. Compartmental pharmacokinetics and tissue distribution of the antifungal echinocandin lipopeptide micafungin (FK463) in rabbits. Antimicrob Agents Chemother 2001;45:3322–7.
[62] Petraitis V, Petraitiene R, Groll AH, et al. Comparative antifungal activities and plasma pharmacokinetics of micafungin (FK463) against disseminated candidiasis and invasive pulmonary aspergillosis in persistently neutropenic rabbits. Antimicrob Agents Chemother 2002;46:1857–69.
[63] Groll AH, Giri N, Petraitis V, et al. Comparative efficacy and distribution of lipid formulations of amphotericin B in experimental *Candida albicans* infection of the central nervous system. J Infect Dis 2000;182:274–82.

ELSEVIER
SAUNDERS

INFECTIOUS
DISEASE CLINICS
OF NORTH AMERICA

Infect Dis Clin N Am 19 (2005) 617–628

Fluoroquinolone Antibiotics in Infants and Children

Urs B. Schaad, MD

Department of Pediatrics, University Children's Hospital UKBB, Römergasse 8, 4058 Basel, Switzerland

Despite class label warnings against use in children, prescriptions for quinolone antibiotics to treat infections in children have become increasingly prevalent. Many of the characteristics of the contemporary fluoroquinolones, the derivatives of the first quinolone antibiotic, nalidixic acid, are particularly appealing for certain pediatric populations. The fluoroquinolones are rapidly bactericidal and have an extended antimicrobial spectrum that includes *Pseudomonas,* gram-positive cocci, and intracellular pathogens. They have advantageous pharmacokinetic properties, such as absorption from the gastrointestinal tract, excellent penetration into many tissues, and good intracellular diffusion. These antimicrobials have been effective in the treatment or prevention of a variety of bacterial infections in adults, including infections of the respiratory and urinary tracts, skin and soft tissue, bone and joint, and eye and ear. Overall, fluoroquinolones are generally well tolerated; the most frequent adverse events during treatment are gastrointestinal disturbances, reactions of the central nervous system, and skin reactions [1,2].

The use of fluoroquinolones in children has been limited because of their potential to induce arthropathy in juvenile animals [3–5]. This extraordinary form of age-related drug toxicity has been shown with all the fluoroquinolones tested so far and has led to important restrictions: Their use has been considered to be contraindicated in children, in growing adolescents, and in women during pregnancy and lactation. Since the mid-1980s, many children have received treatment with fluoroquinolones (mainly ciprofloxacin), however, because they are the only oral antimicrobials with potential activity against such multiply resistant and difficult-to-treat infections as *Pseudomonas aeruginosa* infections in children with cystic fibrosis, complicated urinary tract infections, and enteric infections in developing countries. Results of these trials indicate that prolonged therapy with the fluoroquinolones is effective

E-mail address: urs-b.schaad@unibas.ch

doi:10.1016/j.idc.2005.05.005 **id.theclinics.com**

and well tolerated in pediatric patients, with no significant evidence of arthropathy, bone abnormalities, or other serious adverse events [6]. Besides feared arthrotoxicity, the second major concern regarding use of fluoroquinolones in children is the potential impact on bacterial resistance development [6].

Quinolone arthropathy

History

Soon after the marketing of nalidixic acid in 1962, a child with soreness in one wrist during therapy for urinary tract infection was described [7]. Nalidixic acid was not initially contraindicated in children, but approved for use in children with urinary tract infections in March 1964. Eight years later, another report described a 22-year-old woman who developed severe polyarthritis during a second course of nalidixic acid [8]. These "incapacitating" cases of arthralgia/arthritis were considered as allergic manifestations. Data on file of the manufacturers were cited to contain "about a dozen such reports." These clinical observations with nalidixic acid prompted experimental exposure of laboratory animals to quinolone compounds. The first observations of quinolone-induced cartilage toxicity made with nalidixic, oxolinic, and pipemidic acid administration to young beagle dogs were reported by Ingham et al in 1977 [9], Tatsumi et al in 1978 [10], and Gough et al in 1979 [3].

Use of nalidixic acid in children

Four groups performed a retrospective matched control search for cartilage toxicity in pediatric patients who had received nalidixic acid therapy, in most cases for acute or recurrent urinary tract infections [11–14]. Details of patients and therapies are shown in Table 1. History of symptoms and clinical/radiologic examinations compatible with possible arthropathies

Table 1
Retrospective matched control search for cartilage toxicity in nalidixic acid–treated pediatric patients: details of patients and therapies

Investigators, country	Year of report	No. patient pairs	Age at therapy (y)[a]	Duration of Nalidixic acid therapy (d)[a]	Follow-up time (y)[a]
Schaad, et al Switzerland [11]	1987	11	0.3–9.6 (1.4)	9–600 (17)	3–12 (8)
Rumler and von Rodhden, Germany [12]	1987	201	1–7.2 (6.5)	27–1689 (168)	≥2
Adam, Germany [13]	1989	50	0.1–11 (4.8)	10–815 (118)	≥2
Nuutinen et al, Finland [14]	1994	39	0.3–10.1 (5.3)	6–570 (86)	15–25 (20)

[a] Ranges (mean value).

was recorded, and at follow-up examination growth curves and functional and radiologic joint findings were obtained. The results were similar in the index and control cases. All reports concluded that nalidixic acid does not cause arthropathy in children, even after long-term and high-dose therapy.

Animal experiments

All quinolones tested, including the older compounds and the newer derivatives, have been shown to induce changes in immature cartilage of weight-bearing joints in all laboratory animals tested (mice, rats, dogs, marmosets, guinea pigs, rabbits, and ferrets) [2,4,5,15]. Quinolone-induced arthropathy is limited to juvenile animals except when pefloxacin has been used. Juvenile dogs are generally more sensitive to the arthropathic effects of quinolones than are other species. Healing of quinolone-induced arthropathy is incomplete even after complete clinical recovery; structural changes are at least in part irreversible.

Typical histopathologic lesions after quinolone exposure include fluid-filled blisters, fissures, erosions, and clustering of chondrocytes, usually accompanied by noninflammatory joint effusion. Under the electron microscope, necrosis of the chondrocytes and swelling of the mitochondria are observed initially, followed by disruption of extracellular matrix [16]. Loss of collagen and glycosaminoglycan is an early sequela to the degeneration of chondrocytes [17]. When clinically manifested, the quinolone-induced joint lesions present as acute arthritis, including limping and swelling. The specific mechanism responsible for the initiation of quinolone-induced arthropathy has not been determined. At present, inhibition of mitochondrial DNA replication [18] and the role of magnesium deficiency [19,20] are the most discussed hypotheses.

Neither pharmacokinetic nor pharmacodynamic data can explain the variable arthropathic "power" of different compounds. There also is no clear effect of the molecular structure of the given compound regarding its cartilage toxicity (e.g., quinolones that are fluorinated versus quinolones that are not fluorinated).

Possible monitoring for quinolone-induced cartilage toxicity in patients

The available methods for monitoring for quinolone-induced cartilage toxicity are the following:

- Histopathology—the gold standard [21]
- MRI—the parameters are surface, thickness, and structure of cartilage; presence of effusion (especially recessus suprapatellaris); and bone/cartilage integrity [22–24]; predictive value of MRI has been shown in studies with rabbits, pigs, and dogs [25]
- Sonography—measurement includes presence/absence of effusion and thickness and surface of cartilage [23–26]

- Clinical examination—indicating symptoms and signs would be arthralgia, limping, and joint swelling and for long-term follow-up growth rate; in many animal experiments, cartilage toxicity was documented without any clinical manifestation

Review of published data

A comprehensive review of published reports including monitoring for quinolone-induced cartilage toxicity in patients was performed [27–32]. The reviewed studies included all case reports of suspected quinolone-associated arthralgia/arthropathy in children and adolescents and all multipatient studies on the use of quinolone compounds in skeletally immature patients (open-label and controlled trials) in which there were data on safety, especially regarding potential arthropathy. Most of the data were based on clinical findings—musculoskeletal complaints and joint examination. Such findings do not allow one to distinguish between coincidental joint problems and quinolone-induced arthropathy. As outlined before, only rarely MRI, ultrasonography, and growth curve have been used for either short-term or long-term evaluation. With the exception of the findings in two cystic fibrosis patients [21], the gold standard parameter "histopathology" is lacking. There are four conclusions:

1. To date, there is no unequivocal documentation of quinolone-induced arthropathy in patients as described in juvenile animals; quinolone arthropathy remains an experimental laboratory phenomenon in juvenile animals.
2. Clinical observations temporally related to quinolone use are reversible episodes of arthralgia with and without effusions that do not lead to long-term sequelae when treatment with the agents is discontinued.
3. Most joint complaints associated with quinolone use are coincidental and do not represent adverse effects. Possible coincidental conditions include arthropathy and hypertrophic pulmonary osteoarthropathy associated with cystic fibrosis [33] and reactive, traumatic, and rheumatic joint diseases.
4. It is postulated that the so-called allergic arthritis initially described in nalidixic acid–treated patients does exist but is not the same as the quinolone-induced arthropathy in animals. These adverse events are always transient arthralgic or arthritic manifestations, usually involving large joints and occurring during the first and second week of therapy. The overall incidence is 1% to 3% (–18%) depending on the studied patient group and quinolone compound.

Tendinopathy

Other musculoskeletal adverse effects of quinolones are tendinitis and tendon rupture. Clinical information on quinolone-induced tendinopathy is relatively scarce. Review of the literature on fluoroquinolone-associated tendinopathy [34–37] reveals the following. The incidence in a healthy population is very low, especially in children [36]. In most cases, the Achilles tendon is affected with symptoms compatible with painful tendinitis or with rupture—usually occurring during the second week of treatment. Fluoroquinolone-associated tendinopathy increases in patients who have renal dysfunction (hemodialysis, after renal transplantation). There is a correlation between long-term cortical steroid therapy and age 60 years or older; the male-to-female ratio is approximately 2:1.

Development of bacterial resistance

As mentioned before, there is great concern regarding the potential impact of widespread fluoroquinolone use in children on bacterial resistance development [6,15,30,38,39]. Historically, antimicrobial use has led to the development of drug resistance. The relevant drivers are overuse (volume of antibiotic used in humans and in animals), misuse (inappropriate use), clonal spread (global travel, hygiene, hospital, daycare, family, switch of serotypes), and type of antibiotic. Overuse (eg, for viral infection, as prophylaxis, many veterinarian indications) reflects inadequate knowledge of the prescribing physician and unavailability of diagnostic methods. Appropriate use (avoidance of misuse) includes not only classic selection of an optimal, antibiotic but also individual optimization of dosage and duration of therapy. Well-defined antibiotic policies, good hygiene measures, and strong infection control programs represent key points for limiting the spread of antibiotic resistance.

Bacteria can become resistant to quinolones by mutations in the target molecules (gyrase protein, topoisomerase) or by active drug efflux. With regard to quinolone resistance, great variations exist between bacterial species, clinical settings, and local epidemiology. Resistance is the phenotypic expression corresponding to genetic changes caused by either mutation or acquisition of new genetic information. In some cases, multidrug resistance occurs. *Streptococcus pneumoniae* is one of the most important respiratory pathogens, playing a major role in upper and lower respiratory tract infections. Pneumococcal resistance to antimicrobials may be acquired by means of horizontal transfer followed by homologous recombination of genetic material from the normal flora of the human oral cavity or by means of mutation. Resistance in pneumococci to penicillins and macrolides has been increasing for some time, but more recently fluoroquinolone resistance has become an issue as well [40,41]. Fluoroquinolone resistance is not limited to *S pneumoniae* and has been documented in other pathogens, including those responsible for urinary, respiratory, and gastrointestinal tract infections; skin and soft tissue and bone and joint infections; sexually transmitted diseases; and ulcers [38,39].

Evidence is accumulating that multidrug resistance in pneumococci is related to prescription of antimicrobial agents to a crucial reservoir of these organisms—children. This multidrug resistance likely occurs because children, more often than adults, are colonized with high-density populations of pneumococci in the nasopharynx, which increases the potential for resistance development [38]. Supporting this concern are studies of daycare centers and pediatric long-term care centers that have found a very high prevalence of nasopharyngeal carriage of drug-resistant strains of *S pneumoniae* [42,43]. Overcrowding facilitates the transmission of resistance strains from colonized to susceptible infants and children, who serve as a source for further transmission to family members and ultimately to the general population [44].

A new concern about widespread use of fluoroquinolones to treat children and adults is the recognition of horizontal transfer of fluoroquinolone resistance from viridans group streptococci (eg, *S oralis* and *S mitis*) to *S pneumoniae* [45,46]. When resistance mutations develop in these naturally commensal organisms as a result o fluoroquinolone exposure (even in the absence of pathogenic pneumococci), any subsequent pneumococcal infection carries the risk that the infecting strain of *S pneumoniae* will readily acquire fluoroquinolone resistance–determining DNA regions when antimicrobial therapies are instituted. These fluoroquinolone-resistant *S pneumoniae* can be spread easily from child to parent, followed by widespread dissemination to the adult population. The dangerous triad of antibiotic overuse and misuse, a reservoir of resistant genes, and a closed-space pneumococcal infection (eg, otitis media) could come together with widespread, uncontrolled use of fluoroquinolones in pediatric patients [38].

Pharmacology

The pharmacokinetic data on fluoroquinolones in pediatric patients are limited, and for neonatal patients, the data are anecdotal only [47–51]. The results of available studies, most of which were conducted in cystic fibrosis patients, indicate that systemic clearance is increased in young children; this has led to recommendations for higher doses as shown in Table 2. In

Table 2
Current dosage recommendations

Drug	Route	Dose (mg/kg)	No. doses/day	Maximum daily dose (mg)
Ciprofloxacin	PO	15–20	2	1500
	IV	10–15	2	800
Ofloxacin[a]	PO	7.5	2	800
	IV	5	2	600
Norfloxacin[b]	PO	10–15	2	800

[a] Most pediatric experience in cystic fibrosis patients.
[b] Most pediatric experience in urinary tract infections.

general, fluoroquinolones are absorbed rapidly from the gastrointestinal tract. The range for bioavailability is vast, however, with norfloxacin being 10% to 30% and ofloxacin 80% to 90%. All of the newer compounds except norfloxacin have excellent tissue and intracellular penetration at the recommended therapeutic doses. Quinolones generally are excreted either predominantly in the urine (often as parent compound) or through the bile, in which some undergo enterohepatic recirculation.

Potential indications

Established use

Since the mid-1980s, fluoroquinolones have been used in pediatric patients primarily in circumstances where they were the only antimicrobial choice for infections caused by multiply-resistant organisms [6,15,30]. These included pseudomonal infections in children with cystic fibrosis [23,26,31,51,52], complicated urinary tract infections [53,54], enteric infections in developing countries [27,55,56], and chronic ear infections [57]. Results of controlled clinical trials in patients with these four indications have shown comparable efficacy of the fluoroquinolones and conventional regimens.

Preliminary experience in pediatric patients also indicates that the fluoroquinolones are effective and safe for the prevention or therapy of infections in neutropenic cancer patients [58,59] and for the eradication of nasopharyngeal carriage of meningococci [60]. Fluoroquinolones also have been used successfully when severe infections, including meningitis during the neonatal period, are due to enterobacteria resistance to standard treatment [32,61].

Future use

Research on chemical modifications of the quinolones has been aimed at (1) more potent derivatives, (2) less frequent resistance, (3) better penetration into cerebrospinal fluid, and (4) improved patient tolerability. Some of the newer compounds have achieved many of these goals.

Of major interest for pediatricians are the effective cerebrospinal fluid penetration and the excellent in vitro activity of the new fluoroquinolones against the pathogens that commonly cause bacterial meningitis in children older than 3 months of age, including strains of *S pneumoniae* resistant to β-lactams and to other antibiotics. Based on efficacy data in experimental animals and good cerebrospinal fluid penetration data in humans, a large multicenter, randomized, clinical trial was conducted in children with bacterial meningitis to compare the safety and efficacy of trovafloxacin with that of ceftriaxone with or without vancomycin therapy [62]. This study was terminated earlier than planned because of concerns regarding potential, life-threatening liver toxicity associated with the use of trovafloxacin in adults with severe infections. Of the initially planned 284 children to be evaluable, only 203 (71%) were available for analysis at the time of trial closure. Although optimal statistical power required to draw firm conclusions was not reached, study results suggested that trovafloxacin is therapeutically equivalent to ceftriaxone with or without vancomycin for the management of bacterial meningitis in infants and children. Rates of bacterial eradication, cure, severe sequelae, and death were similar for both treatment groups at the end of treatment and at follow-up assessments. Future trials with other new fluoroquinolone compounds are warranted in pediatric patients with meningitis, but they will be difficult to conduct in view of the risk of rare side effects and possible treatment delays, which are a more important factor than resistance in the occurrence of sequelae.

Other potential future uses of newer fluoroquinolone compounds include childhood otitis media [63]. Increased resistance of pneumococci and other pathogens to available antibiotics raises concerns about bacteriologic and clinical failure in children with acute otitis media. Few therapeutic options exist for patients with recurrent infections or recent treatment failure. The good efficacy of the fluoroquinolone gatifloxacin in pediatric patients with refractory acute otitis media was shown in two trials [64,65]. For recurrent otitis media and otitis media treatment failure, the new fluoroquinolones seem to fill an unmet need.

Summary

The two major concerns regarding use of fluoroquinolones in children are development of bacterial resistance and cartilage toxicity as described in juvenile animals. The risk for rapid emergence of resistance among pneumococci and other common bacterial pathogens, associated with widespread, uncontrolled use of fluoroquinolones in pediatric patients, is a realistic threat. Cartilage toxicity with fluoroquinolones is a laboratory phenomenon in juvenile animals, and no arthropathy has been documented unequivocally in the large numbers of children treated with these agents. Nevertheless, expectant observation is warranted for any new quinolone use in pediatric patients.

Based on available data showing the safety and efficacy of the fluoroquinolones, selected pediatric patients should not be deprived of the therapeutic advantages that these agents have to offer. The quinolones should never be used in pediatric patients for routine treatment, however, when alternative safe and effective antimicrobials are known. To date, established pediatric indications for the fluoroquinolones include bronchopulmonary exacerbation in cystic fibrosis, complicated urinary tract infection, invasive gastrointestinal infection, and chronic ear infection. Potential pediatric indications are bacterial meningitis and refractory acute otitis media.

In most countries, fluoroquinolones so far are approved for use only in pediatric patients with cystic fibrosis and complicated urinary tract infection.

Authorization for broader use of new fluoroquinolones in children must combine efforts of experts in microbiology and infectious diseases, regulatory authorities, and pharmaceutical manufacturers. Postmarketing surveillance must include an adequate risk management plan feasible for patients, parents, and drug companies.

The fluoroquinolones must continue to serve mainly for second-line use in children, only after failure of an earlier treatment and when other antibiotics approved for pediatrics cannot be used. These guidelines would ensure that these agents remain effective for selected infants and children with difficult-to-treat infections.

References

[1] Stahlmann R. Safety profile of the quinolones. J Antimicrob Chemother 1990;26(Suppl D): 31–44.

[2] Stahlmann R, Lode H. The quinolones—safety overview: toxicity, adverse events, and drug interactions. In: Andriole VT, editor. The quinolones. London: Academic Press; 1988. p. 201–3.

[3] Gough A, Barsoum NJ, Mitchell L, McGuire EJ, de la Iglesia FA. Juvenile canine drug-induced arthropathy: clinicopathological studies on articular lesions caused by oxolinic and pipemidic acids. Toxicol Appl Pharmacol 1979;51:177–87.

[4] Christ W, Lehnert T, Ulbrich B. Specific toxicologic aspects of the quinolones. Rev Infect Dis 1988;10(Suppl 1):141–6.

[5] Schluter G. Ciprofloxacin: toxicologic evaluation of additional safety data. Am J Med 1989; 87(Suppl 5A):37–9.

[6] Schaad UB, Salam MA, Aujard Y, et al. Use of fluoroquinolones in pediatrics: consensus report of an International Society of Chemotherapy commission. Pediatr Infect Dis J 1995; 14:1–9.

[7] McDonald DF, Short HB. Usefulness of nalidixic acid in treatment of urinary tract infections. Antimicrob Agents Chemother 1964;64:628–31.

[8] Bailey RR, Natale R, Linton AL. Nalidixic acid arthralgia. Can Med Assoc J 1972;107: 604–7.

[9] Ingham B, Brentnall DW, Dale EA, McFadzean JA. Arthropathy induced by antibacterial fused n-alkyl-4-pyrodoine-3-carboxylic acids. Toxicol Lett 1977;1:21–6.

[10] Tatsumi H, Senda H, Yatera S, Takemoto Y, Yamayoshi M, Onishi K. Toxicological studies on pipedimic acid: V. effect on diarthrodial joints of experimental animals. J Toxicol Sci 1978;3:357–67.

[11] Schaad UB, Wedgwood-Krucko J. Nalidixic acid in children: retrospective matched controlled study for cartilage toxicity. Infection 1987;15:165–8.

[12] Rumler W, von Rodhden L. Does nalidixic acid produce joint toxicity in childhood? In: Book of Abstracts of the 15th International Congress of Chemotherapy, Istanbul, Turkey; 1987. p. 1029–31.

[13] Adam D. Use of quinolone in pediatric patients. Rev Infect Dis 1989;11(Suppl 5):S1113–6.

[14] Nuutinen M, Turtinen J, Uhari M. Growth and joint symptoms in children treated with nalidixic acid. Pediatr Infect Dis J 1994;13:798–800.

[15] Schaad UB. Use of the quinolones in pediatrics. In: Andriole VT, editor. The Quinolones. 3rd ed. San Diego: Academic Press; 2000. p. 455–75.

[16] Stahlmann R, Merker HJ, Hinz N, Chahoud I, Webb J, Neubert D. Ofloxacin in juvenile non-human primates and rats: arthropathia and drug plasma concentrations. Arch Toxicol 1990;64:193–204.

[17] Burkhardt JE, Hill MA, Carlton WW. Morphologic and biochemical changes in articular cartilages of immature beagle dogs dosed with difloxacin. Toxicol Pathol 1992;20:246–52.
[18] Kato M, Takada S, Ogawara S, Takayama S. Effect of levofloxacin on glycosaminoglycan and DNA synthesis of cultured rabbit chondrocytes at concentrations inducing cartilage lesions in vivo. Antimicrob Agents Chemother 1995;39:1979–83.
[19] Forster C, Kociok K, Shakibaei M, et al. Integrins on joint cartilage chondrocytes and alterations by ofloxacin or magnesium deficiency in immature rats. Arch Toxicol 1996;70: 261–70.
[20] Vormann J, Forster C, Zippel U, et al. Effects of magnesium deficiency on magnesium calcium content in bone and cartilage in developing rats in correlation to chondrotoxicity. Calcif Tissue Int 1997;61:230–8.
[21] Schaad UB, Sander E, Wedgwood J, Schaffner T. Morphologic studies for skeletal toxicity after prolonged ciprofloxacin therapy in two juvenile cystic fibrosis patients. Pediatr Infect Dis J 1992;11:1047–9.
[22] Schaad UB, Stoupis C, Wedgwood J, Tschaeppeler H, Vock P. Clinical, radiologic and magnetic resonance monitoring for skeletal toxicity in pediatric patients with cystic fibrosis receiving a three-month course of ciprofloxacin. Pediatr Infect Dis J 1991;10:723–9.
[23] Richard DA, Nousia-Arvanitakis S, Sollich V, Hampel B, Sommerauer B, Schaad UB, and the Cystic Fibrosis Study Group. Oral ciprofloxacin versus intravenous ceftazidime plus tobramycin in pediatric cystic fibrosis patients: comparison of antipseudomonas efficacy and assessment of safety using ultrasonography and magnetic resonance imaging. Pediatr Infect Dis J 1997;16:572–8.
[24] Arico M, Bossi G, Caselli D, et al. Long-term magnetic resonance survey of cartilage damage in leukemic children treated with fluoroquinolones. Pediatr Infect Dis 1995;14:713–4.
[25] Gylys-Morin VM, Hajek PC, Sartoris DJ, Resnick D. Articular cartilage defects: detectability in cadaver knees with MR. Am J Radiol 1987;148:1153–7.
[26] Church DA, Kanga JF, Kuhn RF, et al. Sequential ciprofloxacin therapy in pediatric cystic fibrosis: comparative study vs. ceftazidime/tobramycin in the treatment of acute pulmonary exacerbations. Pediatr Infect Dis J 1997;16:97–105.
[27] Pradhan KM, Arora NK, Jena A, Susheela AK, Bhan MK. Safety of ciprofloxacin therapy in children: magnetic resonance images, body fluid levels of fluoride and linear growth. Acta Paediatr 1995;84:555–60.
[28] Bethell DB, Hien TT, Phi LT, et al. Effects on growth of single short courses of fluoroquinolones. Arch Dis Child 1996;74:44–6.
[29] Burkhardt JE, Walterspiel JN, Schaad UB. Quinolone arthropathy in animals versus children. Clin Infect Dis 1997;25:1196–204.
[30] Gendrel D, Chalumeau M, Moulin F, Raymond J. Fluoroquinolones in paediatrics: a risk for the patient or for the community? Lancet Infect Dis 2003;3:537–46.
[31] Chalumeau M, Tonnelier S, d'Athis P, et al. Fluoroquinolone safety in pediatric patients: a prospective, multicenter, comparative cohort study in France. Pediatrics 2003;111: e714–9.
[32] Drosso-Agakidou V, Roilides E, Papakyriakidou-Koliouska P, et al. Use of ciprofloxacin in neonatal sepsis: lack of adverse effects up to one year. Pediatr Infect Dis J 2004;23:346–9.
[33] Phillips BB, David T. Pathogenesis and management of arthropathy in cystic fibrosis. J R Soc Med 1996;79(Suppl 12):44–50.
[34] van der Linden PD, van de Lei J, Nab HW, Knol A, Stricker BH. Achilles tendinitis associated with fluoroquinolones. Br J Clin Pharmacol 1999;48:433–7.
[35] van der Linden PD, Sturkenboom MCJM, Herings RMC, Leufkens HGM, Stricker BH. Fluoroquinolones and risk of Achilles tendon disorders: case-control study. BMJ 2002;324: 1306–7.
[36] Yee CL, Duffy C, Gerbino PG, Stryker S, Noel GJ. Tendon or joint disorders in children after treatment with fluoroquinolones or azithromycin. Pediatr Infect Dis J 2002;21: 525–9.

[37] Khaliq Y, Zhanel GG. Fluoroquinolone-associated tendinopathy: a critical review of the literature. Clin Infect Dis 2003;36:1404–10.
[38] Mandell LA, Peterson LR, Wise R, et al. The battle against emerging antibiotic resistance: should fluoroquinolones be used to treat children? Clin Infect Dis 2002;35:721–7.
[39] Hooper DC. New uses for new and old quinolones and the challenge of resistance. Clin Infect Dis 2000;30:243–54.
[40] Chen DK, McGeer A, De Azavedo JC, Low DE. Decreased susceptibility of *Streptococcus pneumoniae* to fluoroquinolones in Canada. N Engl J Med 1999;341:233–9.
[41] Ho PL, Yung RW, Tsang DN, et al. Increasing resistance of *Streptococcus pneumoniae* to fluoroquinolones: results of a Hong Kong multicentre study in 2000. J Antimicrob Chemother 2001;48:659–65.
[42] Yagupsky P, Porat N, Fraser D, et al. Acquisition, carriage, and transmission of pneumococci with decreased antibiotic susceptibility in young children attending a day care facility in southern Israel. J Infect Dis 1998;177:1003–12.
[43] Mannheimer SB, Riley LW, Roberts RB. Association of penicillin-resistant pneumococci with residence in a pediatric chronic care facility. J Infect Dis 1996;174:513–9.
[44] Kronenberger CB, Hoffmann RE, Lezotte DC, Marine WM. Invasive penicillin-resistant pneumococcal infections: a prevalence and historical cohort study. Emerg Infect Dis 1996;2: 121–4.
[45] Gonzales J, Georgiou M, Alcaide F, Balas D, Linares J, de la Campa AG. Fluoroquinolone resistance mutations in the parC, parE, and gyrA genes of clinical isolates of viridans group streptococci. Antimicrob Agents Chemother 1998;42:2792–8.
[46] Ferrandiz MJ, Fernoll A, Linares J, de la Campa AG. Horizontal transfer of parC and gyrA in fluoroquinolone-resistant clinical isolates of *Streptococcus pneumoniae*. Antimicrob Agents Chemother 2000;44:840–7.
[47] Blumer JL, Stern RC, Myers CM, et al. Pharmacokinetics and pharmacodynamics of ciprofloxacin in cystic fibrosis. Abstracts of 14th Internationl Congress on Chemotherapy, Kyoto, 1985.
[48] Stutman HR, Shalit I, Marks MI, Greenwood R, Chartrand SA, Hillman BC. Pharmacokinetics of two dosage regimens of ciprofloxacin during a two-week-therapeutic trial in patients with cystic fibrosis. Am J Med 1987;82(Suppl 4A):142–5.
[49] Peltola H, Vaarala M, Renkonen O, Neuvonen PJ. Pharmacokinetics of single dose of oral ciprofloxacin in infants and small children. Antimicrob Agents Chemother 1992;36: 1086–90.
[50] Schaeffer HG, Strass H, Wedgwood J, et al. Pharmacokinetics of ciprofloxacin in pediatric cystic fibrosis patients. Antimicrob Agents Chemother 1996;40:29–34.
[51] Rubio TT, Miles MV, Lettiere JT, Kuhn RJ, Echols RM, Church DA. Pharmacokinetic disposition of sequential intravenous/oral ciprofloxacin in pediatric cystic fibrosis patients with acute pulmonary exacerbation. Pediatr Infect Dis J 1997;16:112–7.
[52] Schaad UB, Wedgwood J, Ruedeberg A, Kraemer R, Hampel B. Ciprofloxacin as antipseudomonal treatment in patients with cystic fibrosis. Pediatr Infect Dis J 1997;16: 106–11.
[53] Fujii R. The use of norfloxacin in children in Japan. Adv Antineopl Chemother 1992;11: 219–32.
[54] Koyle MA, Barqawi A, Wild J, Passamaneck M, Furness PD. Pediatric urinary tract infections: the role of fluoroquinolones. Pediatr Infect Dis J 2003;22:1133–7.
[55] Green S, Tillotson G. Use of ciprofloxacin in developing countries. Pediatr Infect Dis J 1997; 16:150–9.
[56] Salam MA, Dhar U, Khan WA, Bennish ML. Randomised comparison of ciprofloxacin suspension and pivmecillinam for childhood shigellosis. Lancet 1998;352:522–7.
[57] Lang R, Goshen S, Raas-Rothschild A. Oral ciprofloxacin in the management of chronic suppurative otitis media without cholesteatoma in children. Pediatr Infect Dis J 1992;11: 925–9.

[58] Freifeld A, Pizzo P. Use of fluoroquinolones for empirical management of febrile neutropenia in pediatric cancer patients. Pediatr Infect Dis J 1997;16:140–6.
[59] Patrick CC. Use of fluoroquinolones as prophylaxis agents in patients with neutropenia. Pediatr Infect Dis J 1997;16:135–9.
[60] Cuevas LE, Kazembe P, Mughogho GK, Tilloston GS, Hart CA. Eradication of nasopharyngeal carriage of *Neisseria meningitidis* in children and adult in rural Africa: a comparision of ciprofloxacin and rifampicin. J Infect Dis 1995;171:728–31.
[61] Krcmery V, Filka J, Uher J, et al. Ciprofloxacin in treatment of nosocomial meningitis in neonates and in infants: report of 12 cases and review. Diag Microbiol Infect Dis 1999;35: 75–80.
[62] Saez-Llorens X, Mccoig C, Feris JM, et al. Quinolone treatment for pediatric bacterial meningitis: a comparative study of trovafloxacin and ceftriaxone with or without vancomycin. Pediatr Infect Dis J 2002;21:14–22.
[63] Dagan R, Arguedas A, Schaad UB. Potential role of fluoroquinolone therapy in childhood otitis media. Pediatr Infect Dis J 2004;23:390–8.
[64] Leibovitz E, Piglansky L, Raiz S, et al. Bacteriologic and clinical efficacy of oral gatifloxacin for the treatment of recurrent/nonresponsive acute otitis media: an open label, non-comparative, double tymopanocentesis study. Pediatr Infect Dis J 2003;22:943–9.
[65] Arguedas A, Sher L, Lopez E, et al. Open label, multicenter study of gatifloxacin treatment of recurrent otitis media and acute otitis media treatment failure. Pediatr Infect Dis J 2003; 22:949–55.

ELSEVIER
SAUNDERS

INFECTIOUS
DISEASE CLINICS
OF NORTH AMERICA

Infect Dis Clin N Am 19 (2005) 629–645

The Epidemiology of Childhood Pneumococcal Disease in the United States in the Era of Conjugate Vaccine Use

Philip Toltzis, MD[a,*], Michael R. Jacobs, MD, PhD[b]

[a]*Department of Pediatrics, Rainbow Babies and Children's Hospital, Case Western Reserve University School of Medicine, 11100 Euclid Avenue, Cleveland, OH 44102, USA*

[b]*Department of Pathology, University Hospitals of Cleveland, Case Western Reserve University School of Medicine, 11100 Euclid Avenue, Cleveland, OH 44102, USA*

In February 2000, a heptavalent pneumococcal conjugate vaccine (PCV7 [Prevnar]) was licensed in the United States for administration to children younger than 5 years of age. The development of this vaccine was prompted by the observation that young children, especially children younger than 2 years old, were disproportionately affected by serious pneumococcal infection, and by the recognition that the available 23-valent polysaccharide vaccine was largely nonimmunogenic in this population. Soon after the licensure of PCV7, the Centers for Disease Control and Prevention (CDC)–sponsored Advisory Committee on Immunization Practices [1] and the American Academy of Pediatrics Committee on Infectious Diseases [2] recommended universal immunization for children younger than 24 months of age, with a schedule composed of three doses given at 2-month intervals between age 2 and 6 months and a booster dose at 12 to 15 months. Additionally, immunization with the conjugate vaccine (coupled with subsequent administration of the 23-valent polysaccharide vaccine) was recommended for children age 2 to 5 years at high risk for serious pneumococcal infection. Shortages of vaccine were encountered shortly after these recommendations were made and have persisted since [3]. Despite this situation, the pediatric community rapidly embraced the universal pneumococcal immunization program, and receipt of at least three doses in the eligible population approached 70% by 2003 [4,5].

* Corresponding author.
E-mail address: pxt2@case.edu (P. Toltzis).

0891-5520/05/$ - see front matter
doi:10.1016/j.idc.2005.05.008
id.theclinics.com

The conjugate vaccine was designed to include the seven serotypes most responsible for infection in young American children—4, 6B, 9V, 14, 18C, 19F, and 23F (hereafter referred to as the *vaccine serotypes*). Before the introduction of the vaccine, these serotypes accounted for approximately 80% of invasive pneumococcal disease and the marked majority of noninvasive disease, particularly otitis media, in the target population [1,6,7]. The same serotypes also were represented prominently among isolates expressing antibiotics resistance [1]. PCV7 contains 2 μg of capsular sugars from each serotype except 6B, of which 4 μg is included. Immunogenicity among young children is enhanced by the binding of the capsular molecules to the carrier protein CRM_{197}, a nontoxic mutation of diphtheria toxin. It was hoped that immunization also would elicit cross-protective immunity to related serotypes, particularly 6A, 9A, and 19A. Also, 9-valent and 11-valent conjugate vaccines have been developed, including additional serotypes that are more common outside the United States, but these have not yet been licensed.

The immunologic response to the 7-valent protein conjugated vaccine has been evaluated by several investigators [8–13]. Geometric mean serum antibody concentrations to each of the seven vaccine serotypes are increased after the second dose. After the third dose, serum antibody concentrations reach or exceed 1 μg/mL for all seven serotypes in nearly all recipients. Titers of antibodies against several of the serotypes decline again by the time the booster dose is administered, but the geometric mean concentrations after boosting range from 3 to 9 μg/mL, with nearly all recipients recording concentrations greater than 1 μg/mL of all vaccine serotypes. The humoral immunologic response is not uniform across serotypes. Selected serotypes (eg, 6B) required more doses to induce a significant response compared with the others. Additionally, the antibody concentrations generated to each serotype vary; post-booster mean geometric concentrations are approximately 2 μg/mL against serotype 4, but greater than 9 μg/mL against serotype 14. The concentration of antibody required for protection for each serotype is unknown, however, and it likely differs from serotype to serotype. In a mouse model of invasive pneumococcal disease, the serum concentration of passively administered antipneumococcal antibody required to reduce mortality by 50% ranged from 0.1 to 3.5 μg/mL depending on the serotype [14]. Similarly, some authors have found a poor correlation between protection against pneumococcal colonization and circulating antipneumococcal antibody concentrations in young children [15].

The effects of universal PCV7 immunization on the epidemiology of pneumococcal disease are not yet fully appreciated, but early results are being reported. This article outlines the impact of this immunization program on pneumococcal colonization and invasive and noninvasive disease, especially in children, and on the occurrence of antibiotic resistance among *Streptococcus pneumoniae*. Factors that may influence the effectiveness of the vaccine in the future also are discussed, particularly the phenomena of herd immunity, serotype replacement, and serotype switching. Finally, the authors examine whether the epidemiology of pneumococcal disease has been sufficiently altered to allow a change in the approach to a febrile child.

Vaccine efficacy

Pneumococcal colonization

Several reports have documented that immunization with conjugate pneumococcal vaccine reduces the incidence of nasopharyngeal carriage by vaccine serotypes [15–20]. These investigations, conducted in Israel, the Gambia, South Africa, and the United States, tested the effects of multiple conjugate vaccine preparations with varying valences administered to different pediatric age groups. Nevertheless, their results were quite similar, documenting that new acquisition of vaccine serotypes is reduced after immunization. Mbelle et al [18] randomized nearly 500 South African children to receive either a 9-valent pneumococcal conjugate vaccine or placebo at 6, 10, and 14 weeks of age. At 9 months of age, carriage of vaccine serotypes was detected in only 18% of vaccine recipients versus 36% of controls ($P < .001$). Likewise, immunization of Israeli toddlers attending daycare centers [16] reduced new colonization by vaccine serotypes on follow-up by 50% ($P < .001$).

Invasive disease

It generally is believed that the invasive capacity of pneumococci is associated strongly with the composition of the capsule, and that only a limited number of serotypes, most of which are contained in the conjugate vaccine, commonly are able to cause invasive disease. A marked beneficial effect of PCV7 on the incidence of invasive disease, primarily bacteremia and meningitis, has been shown repeatedly [5,11,21–29]. The seminal trial reported by investigators from the Northern California Kaiser Permanente group randomized otherwise healthy children to receive either PCV7 or a conjugate meningococcal C vaccine in the late 1990s, before vaccine licensure. This study showed a protective efficacy of greater than 97% against invasive pneumococcal disease from a vaccine serotype in subjects completing the series, results that prompted the early closure of the study [11]. Subsequent analyses by the same group assessed the changes in invasive pneumococcal disease among their roster of more than 3 million people after vaccine licensure [5]. There was a dramatic diminution in invasive pneumococcal disease after the introduction of PCV7 in 2000, most notably among young children [5]. Protection from vaccine and vaccine-related serotypes was nearly universal in children younger than age 2 years. These benefits were documented despite the vaccine shortage experienced shortly after licensure, which precluded administration of the fourth dose in a large proportion of the pediatric cohort.

Most additional reports similarly have compared the incidence of invasive pneumococcal disease in large populations before and after PCV7 licensure. The report from the CDC-sponsored Active Bacterial Core Surveillance network is representative [24]. This network monitored the incidence of invasive pneumococcal disease in seven separate regions in the United States with a combined population of approximately 16 million persons during the years 1996–2001. In children younger than 5 years old, the incidence of invasive pneumococcal infection declined by 59% in 2001, the year after the recommendations for universal immunization were published. As in the Northern California cohort, the reduction was most dramatic in children younger than age 2 years. Among this latter group, the rate of decline was most striking in disease caused by vaccine serotypes, with an aggregate reduction of 78% [24]. Reduction also was noted in disease caused by the principal vaccine-related serotypes (6A, 9A, and 19A), but to a lesser, albeit statistically detectable, degree (rate of reduction 50%). These effects were observed even when the total number of doses sold by the manufacturer indicated incomplete immunization among the study population.

PCV7 has been made available equally to all racial groups in the United States with the result that its protection has been enjoyed across ethnic boundaries [22,27]. In particular, prevaccine disparities in the incidence of invasive pneumococcal disease among African Americans compared with whites have largely disappeared. The black-to-white incidence ratio for invasive pneumococcal disease in children younger than age 2 years was 3.30 during the period before PCV7 licensure and had decreased markedly (1.58) by 2002 [22]. In the years immediately after the recommendation for universal immunization was adopted, the incidence of invasive disease caused by vaccine serotypes decreased 92% among young African-American children [22].

The conjugate vaccine also confers protection against invasive disease in HIV-infected children. This finding is particularly noteworthy because previous studies have failed to show protection by the 23-valent polysaccharide pneumococcal vaccine in HIV-infected adults [30]. Klugman et al [23] employed a 9-valent conjugate vaccine in more than 39,000 children in Soweto, South Africa (three doses at 6, 10, and 14 weeks of age), and measured its protective efficacy by comparing the incidence of disease with that observed in a control group immunized with the *Haemophilus influenzae* type b conjugate vaccine. In the subgroup of HIV-infected children, protection against disease caused by all serotypes was 53%, with an efficacy of 65% recorded for infection caused by a vaccine serotype. This latter statistic was lower than the 83% efficacy recorded for HIV-negative children, but still highly significant compared with *H influenzae* type b–vaccinated, HIV-positive controls ($P < .006$).

Pneumonia

Assessing the efficacy of the conjugate pneumococcal vaccine in preventing pediatric pneumococcal pneumonia is hampered by the inherent uncertainty in identifying the infecting organism in pneumonic disease in children. Studies using clinically or radiographically confirmed pneumonia as their outcome include many children with disease caused by nonpneumococcal pathogens. These limitations notwithstanding, the investigators at the Northern California Kaiser Permanente group attempted to estimate vaccine efficacy in reducing pneumonia by identifying cases through their clinical databases in children randomized to receive PCV7 in their prelicensure trial [31]. Among children who had completed the series, the incidence of pneumonia was reduced by 20.5% (8.7 cases per 1000 person-years versus 11 cases per 1000 person-years in control subjects). Benefit of vaccine was statistically detectable only in children whose pneumonia occurred before their second birthday [31]. In the Soweto trial involving HIV-infected and non–HIV-infected children, the 9-valent vaccine was effective in reducing radiographically documented pneumonia by 17% among vaccine recipients ($P < .01$) [23]. Protective efficacy in HIV-infected children specifically was 13%; however, this value was not statistically significant.

Acute otitis media

Before the introduction of the conjugate pneumococcal vaccine, most cases of acute otitis media (AOM) in childhood were caused by pneumococcus, and most of these were due to vaccine serotypes [32]. Two prospective, randomized, blinded studies including large numbers of subjects assessed the efficacy of vaccine in reducing AOM in children in Finland [33] and in Northern California [34]. Both studies were completed in the mid to late 1990s, before the vaccine was available to the general public. Although designed differently, the vaccine efficacy recorded in the two trials was similar, indicating an efficacy against AOM from any cause of 6% and 7.8% in the Finnish and California studies [33,34]. The reduction in the former trial failed to reach statistical significance. In the Finnish trial, where all episodes of AOM were evaluated by culture of middle ear fluid, vaccine reduced AOM caused by all pneumococci by 34%, by pneumococci of vaccine serotypes by 57%, and by pneumococci of vaccine-related serotypes by 51% [33]. The study end point (diagnosis of AOM) in the Northern California trial was determined through computerized records of visit diagnoses. The data generated suggested that protection from PCV7 against AOM was reduced if fewer than three doses of vaccine were received, and that effectiveness against AOM waned after children reached 2 years of age. Immunization appeared particularly effective in decreasing the number of children affected with recurrent episodes of AOM, with an associated reduction in the need for myringotomy tubes [34].

Dutch investigators [35] completed a trial testing whether PCV7 followed by immunization with the 23-valent pneumococcal polysaccharide vaccine could decrease the frequency of AOM in children who already had an established history of recurrent middle ear infection. In contrast to previous AOM studies, children 1 to 7 years old were recruited. No reduction in episodes of AOM was detectable compared with a control group of children who received the hepatitis vaccine. The investigators postulated that prior episodes of AOM had damaged the architecture of the middle ear and eustachian tube sufficiently to overshadow any advantage of immunization [35].

AOM is nearly universal in children younger than 3 years old [36], and nearly 20% of all sick ambulatory visits in young children are prompted by AOM [37,38]. Although the overall effectiveness of vaccine in reducing AOM is small relative to the reductions documented for invasive disease, it can been argued that even these modest reductions result in a substantial benefit to the public health.

Cost-effectiveness

The use of conjugate *H influenzae* type b vaccine, which costs $390 million per year in the United States, has been estimated to result in the prevention of $1.3 billion in direct annual costs of treating invasive *H influenzae* type b disease, making this a cost-effective vaccine [39]. PCV7 is one of the most expensive vaccines in wide use, however, accounting for nearly 50% of the cost of the recommended childhood vaccines. When PCV7 was introduced, cost-effectiveness projections based on efficacy data collected by the Northern California Kaiser Permanente prelicensure studies indicated a net cost of $80,000 per life-year saved, assuming that every child in a yearly US birth cohort received vaccine. This net cost was predicated on a birth cohort of 3.8 million children, a vaccine list price of $58 per dose, an assumption of four doses being required to confer efficacy, and approximately 90% efficacy for the vaccine against invasive disease [40].

In 2002, the CDC estimated 40.8% coverage for three or more doses of vaccine in children age 19 to 35 months [41]. Again assuming a birth cohort of 3.8 million, this coverage rate would imply that 1,550,400 children were vaccinated that year. Further assuming that half of these children received four doses and the other half three, at $58 per dose, the cost of vaccine would have been $315 million. Using the 2001 CDC incidence data for invasive pneumococcal disease, there would have been 7144 cases of invasive disease per year before introduction of PCV7 and 2242 cases in 2002. By these calculations, each of the 4902 cases prevented in the birth cohort would have cost nearly $65,000 to prevent, and 316 children would have been immunized for each case prevented. These estimations render the universal PCV7 immunization program cost-effective, although considerably more costly than the universal *H influenzae* type b immunization program and many other preventive health interventions [40].

Influence of PCV7 on the proportion of antibiotic-nonsusceptible pneumococcus

In addition to disproportionately causing invasive and noninvasive infection, some of the vaccine and vaccine-related serotypes (serotypes/groups 6, 9, 14, 19, and 23) also account for most pneumococci expressing decreased susceptibility to penicillin, macrolides, and other commonly employed antibiotics [6,20,42,43]. Universal immunization holds the promise of significantly reducing the proportion of nonsusceptible pneumococci circulating in the community. Some trials, particularly trials measuring the effect of conjugate vaccine on pneumococcal colonization and AOM [15,18,44], have indicated a reduction in the proportion of antibiotic-resistant pneumococci after immunization. Other studies, particularly studies measuring the efficacy of vaccine in invasive disease [23–25,27], have indicated, however, that the proportion of pneumococci expressing antibiotic resistance after the introduction of the vaccine has either changed little or not at all. A survey by Stephens et al [27] recorded a dramatic decrease in the incidence of invasive disease caused by macrolide-resistant pneumococci in Georgia after licensure of PCV7, from 7.7 cases per 100,000 persons in 2000 to 2.9 cases per 100,000 persons in 2002, a 69% reduction. The incidence of invasive disease from all pneumococci, regardless of resistance phenotype, decreased, however, by almost the same proportion (57%).

Some of the beneficial effect of PCV7 immunization on reducing the proportion of pneumococci expressing antibiotic resistance may be offset by the emergence of reduced antibiotic susceptibility in nonvaccine serotypes. Even before the introduction of PCV7, a clone of serotype 35B expressing reduced susceptibility to penicillin had appeared throughout the United States [45]. Similarly, during the years 1998–2001, 19% of middle ear isolates from children from southern Israel were nonvaccine serotypes, and of these, nearly 40% were penicillin nonsusceptible [46]. Most of these latter strains were from serotypes 35B, 33F, 21, and 15 B/C, and similar to the American serotype 35B strain, the organisms within each serotype were largely clonally related. Most of these isolates expressed penicillin resistance in the intermediate range, compared with vaccine serotypes that are more commonly overtly penicillin resistant, and the incidence of coresistance with other agents was lower [46].

Dynamic effects of immunization on pneumococcal epidemiology: implications for future efficacy

Although early trials measuring efficacy of PCV7 have been favorable, several characteristics of the vaccine and pneumococcal epidemiology suggest that these effects may change over time. These include characteristics that may render universal PCV7 immunization more effective and less effective than currently appreciated.

Characteristics that may favor improved efficacy over time

Herd immunity

It has been long appreciated that pneumococcal-colonized children are reservoirs for transmission to other children and to household contacts [47–51]. The decrease in nasopharyngeal colonization by vaccine serotypes resulting from conjugate vaccine administration in children may confer benefits to their nonimmunized contacts through herd immunity. A similar phenomenon was experienced after the licensure of the conjugate *H influenzae* type b vaccine, which similarly reduces *H influenzae* nasopharyngeal colonization [52,53]. Evidence that this phenomenon already may be occurring in pneumococci is strongest in prevaccine versus postvaccine incidence studies of invasive disease, indicating a decrease in invasive pneumococcal infection in largely nonimmunized adult populations since 2000. In the survey by the CDC-sponsored Active Bacterial Core Surveillance program [24], the incidence of invasive disease caused by a vaccine serotype in adults age 20 to 39 years declined by 40% ($P < .001$) after introduction of routine immunization in children compared with nonsignificant changes in the incidence of disease caused by vaccine-related and nonvaccine serotypes. A less dramatic benefit (a decrease of 14%) was recorded in adults 40 to 64 years old. Similar statistics have been reported by the Northern California Kaiser Permanente Group [5] and by the Atlanta site of the Active Bacterial Core Surveillance program [27].

Expanding numbers of immunized children may create sufficient herd immunity that the incidence of AOM would be reduced more substantially than recorded in the currently published trials. Results reported by Block et al [54] assessed the yearly incidence of AOM in their highly immunized pediatric population in northern Kentucky in the 3 years after the introduction of the vaccine. In this study, the incidence of AOM was reduced by 19% after vaccine licensure. This decrease was substantially better than that reported by the Finnish and California studies discussed previously [33,34], both of which were conducted before vaccine was available to the general community and before the effects of herd immunity could be fully enjoyed.

Effect of PCV7 immunization on antibiotic use

An indirect benefit of universal PCV7 immunization may be to allow the reduction of antibiotic administration, stemming from the cumulative decrease in AOM and other respiratory tract illnesses caused by pneumococci. Acquisition of a strain of pneumococcus with reduced susceptibility to penicillin and other antibiotics is strongly associated with recent antibiotic exposure [47,55–57]. To date, only a few studies have examined the effect of conjugate pneumococcal vaccine on antibiotic administration. Dagan et al [58], employing a 9-valent conjugate vaccine, recorded a significant decrease in use of antibiotics among immunized Israeli children attending daycare centers (relative risk for treatment 0.85 [$P = .02$] versus children immunized with a meningococcal conjugate vaccine). The group from the Northern California Kaiser Permanente health care system, who similarly compared children receiving PCV7 with children receiving a meningococcal vaccine, recorded a decrease in antibiotic prescription of nearly 6% in children completing the pneumococcal vaccine series [34]. Given the well-placed public health mandate to reduce the use of antibiotics in ambulatory settings, these modest reductions eventually could have a marked impact on the promotion of antibiotic-resistant phenotypes among pneumococci and other community-acquired pathogens.

Characteristics that may reduce vaccine efficacy over time

Vaccine failure

In many reports to date, the number of children fully immunized in the population under study is unknown, disallowing population-based estimates of vaccine failure. The incidence of such failure, particularly in invasive disease, seems to be low, however. In the initial randomized, blinded trial conducted by the Northern California Kaiser Permanente group [11], nearly 11,000 children were fully immunized with PCV7, and only 1 child experienced invasive pneumococcal disease secondary to a vaccine serotype. In contrast, 39 cases were recorded among an essentially identical number of children who had received the meningococcal vaccine. In the survey by the Pediatric Multicenter Pneumococcal Surveillance Group reporting from 8 large children's hospitals, only 10 children admitted during 2001–2002 who had received three doses of PCV7 and 2 who had received all four doses were identified with invasive disease from a vaccine or vaccine-related serotype [26]. Vaccine failure is more common in AOM. Of the 786 PCV7 recipients from the Finnish study with complete immunization and follow-up, a vaccine serotype was isolated from middle ear fluid in 107, and a vaccine-related serotype was isolated in 41 [33].

There is some evidence that the conjugate vaccine may be less protective against disease caused by serogroup 19 compared with the other serogroups represented in the vaccine. Although the incidence of nasopharyngeal colonization [16] and AOM [33,59] from the vaccine-included serotype 19F is reduced after immunization, the degree of reduction is lower compared with that documented for the other vaccine serotypes. Although cross-protection against some vaccine-related serotypes (eg, serotype 6A) is good, cross-protection against the vaccine-related serotype 19A after immunization with 19F capsular polysaccharide has been poor [5,16,23,27,33]. In some studies of invasive disease, there was no detectable change in the incidence of infection secondary to serotype 19A after the licensure of the vaccine [24,27].

Serotype replacement

Chief among concerns of present and continued vaccine efficacy is the phenomenon of serotype replacement—the expansion of colonization and disease from nonvaccine serotypes. Several studies of the effect of conjugate vaccine on nasopharyngeal colonization have documented a significant increase in colonization by nonvaccine serotypes among vaccine recipients versus nonimmunized comparison groups [16,18,19]. In the study by Dagan et al [16], the reduction of colonization by vaccine serotypes in immunized daycare center attendees (overall odds ratio 0.50 compared with controls) was offset by an increased incidence of carriage by nonvaccine serotypes (overall odds ratio 1.59, with an odds ratio of 3.72 among the youngest study group age 15–23 months). Nevertheless, typically carriage of nonvaccine strains tends to be shorter compared with carriage by vaccine serotypes [43], suggesting that a shift toward colonization by the nonvaccine serotypes may be epidemiologically beneficial even if the total incidence of pneumococcal colonization remains largely unaltered.

Serotype replacement also may be relevant in the low vaccine efficacy in AOM. Some of the relatively modest levels of protection against AOM recorded to date have been due to an increasing incidence of AOM caused by nonpneumococcal pathogens, particularly nontypable *H influenzae* [44,59] and the usually rare middle ear pathogen *Staphylococcus aureus* [35,60]. The AOM trial from Finland indicated, however, pneumococcal serotype replacement also was a factor. In this latter study, the reduction in middle ear infection caused by vaccine and vaccine-related pneumococcal serotypes was balanced by an increase of disease caused by nonvaccine serotypes of 33% [33]. Consequently the total reduction of AOM among vaccine recipients was relatively small.

Significant serotype replacement has not been detected in either young children or the total population suffering from blood-borne pneumococcal disease since the introduction of universal PCV7 immunization [5,11, 22,24,27]. Data from the US Pediatric Multicenter Pneumococcal Surveillance Group, which has been monitoring the incidence of pneumococcal infection at their eight tertiary care pediatric hospitals since 1994, reported an increase in invasive disease secondary to nonvaccine serogroups of 28% in 2001 and 66% in 2002, but the absolute number of children affected by disease caused by a nonvaccine serotype remained small [26].

Serotype switching

An additional phenomenon that may confound the future effectiveness of PCV7 is serotype switching—the transformation of vaccine serotype strains to nonvaccine serotypes. Even before introduction of PCV7, strains of pneumococci were identified from daycare centers [61–63] and from national surveys [64] that apparently had switched from one serotype to another. Typically these isolates had identical genetic fingerprint patterns, as established by methods such as pulsed-field gel electrophoresis or random-primer polymerase chain reaction, to strains derived from an alternative serotype and indistinguishable penicillin resistance–associated penicillin-binding proteins and other antibiotic-resistance genes, but the capsule had changed. Exchange of genetic material through transformation occurs regularly in pneumococci in vivo. The genes encoding the capsule in pneumococci reside in a cassette that is flanked by conserved sequences, facilitating the recombination of capsular genes after transformation of bacterial DNA from a co-colonizing strain and the subsequent expression of a new capsular phenotype [65,66]. This phenomenon raises the possibility that vaccine-induced immunity would result in the selection of virulent transformants that have switched to a nonvaccine serotype.

It is uncertain whether serotype switching will be an important factor in determining future vaccine efficacy. The capsular polysaccharides are principal virulence determinants in pneumococci, and switching from an "invasive" serotype to one not usually associated with invasive disease may render the organism less pathogenic. Other virulence factors besides the capsule exist. Experimental transformants that have switched their capsule while retaining the rest of their original genetic background sometimes approximate the virulence of the donor strain and sometimes do not when tested in a mouse model [67]. It is unclear how frequently serotype switching would occur in the age of universal pneumococcal vaccination. McEllistrem et al [68] analyzed isolates from middle ear fluid collected in Pittsburgh during the years spanning the introduction of PCV7. Several instances of serotype switching were identified among these isolates, especially serogroup 19 pneumococci, which had been derived from the worldwide-disseminated Spanish 23F clone. More of these serogroup 19 transformants were isolated after the introduction of the vaccine than before. This study raises the possibility that immunization may select not only nonvaccine serotype transformants, but also serogroup 19 transformants against which PCV7 immunization provides relatively poor protection [68].

Success of PCV7 and the approach to the young febrile child

Given the success of PCV7, particularly in preventing invasive disease, discussions have begun whether to change long-standing approaches to pediatric conditions that traditionally have been caused in large part by pneumococci. Principal among these is the evaluation of a young child with fever of unknown origin [69,70]. Before the introduction of the *H influenzae* and pneumococcal conjugate vaccines, occult bacteremia was noted in 3% to 11% of children age 3 to 36 months with fever greater than 39°C and total white blood cell count of 15,000/mm^3 or more [71,72]. Approximately 10% to 20% of these cases were caused by *H influenzae* type b, and two thirds were caused by pneumococci, with most of the latter due to vaccine-associated serotypes. These observations prompted widely publicized (and frequently debated) guidelines [73] recommending that nontoxic infants with temperature greater than 39°C and no apparent source be evaluated with a complete blood count. In infants whose total white blood cell count exceeded $15{,}000/mm^3$, a single dose of ceftriaxone was recommended after a blood culture was obtained.

Surveys conducted after the introduction of the *H influenzae* type b conjugate vaccine documented that virtually all disease caused by *H influenzae* had been eliminated, and that the incidence of occult bacteremia from all causes had diminished to less than 2%, with greater than 80% of the remaining cases caused by pneumococci [74,75]. To date, only a single retrospective survey of pediatric occult bacteremia has been performed since the introduction of PCV7 [76]. This study recorded only three cases of occult bacteremia (all due to pneumococci) over a 16-month period between late 2001 and 2003 at a large pediatric facility (two of these cases occurred in one child), translating into an incidence of less than 1% [76].

In response to these observations, decision analyses have been performed to determine whether alternative approaches to a nontoxic child with high fever and no source should be pursued in the era of universal *H influenzae* type b and pneumococcal immunization [77,78]. These analyses have considered, among other parameters, the likelihood of permanent injury or death from untreated pneumococcal bacteremia, the risks of adverse reactions to the antibiotic, and the cost incurred by the traditional approach for each prevented case of meningitis or death. Although designed differently, both analyses concluded that careful clinical evaluation and follow-up alone becomes increasingly justified as the incidence of occult bacteremia approaches 0.5% [77,78], a figure likely to be reached given the early reports of vaccine efficacy against invasive pneumococcal disease.

It is still early to judge the long-term effects of PCV7 on the epidemiology of pneumococcal disease in children. Until issues of vaccine failure, especially involving organisms of serogroup 19, serotype replacement, and serotype switching, are fully resolved, it is probably safest to maintain the traditional approach to the evaluation of high fever without source in a young infant [69]. Change in practice ultimately must await prospective trials validating the safety of a less aggressive paradigm. Despite these considerations, a recently published survey [79] indicated that community pediatricians already are less prone to pursue blood testing or administer antibiotics in a febrile infant who had received the PCV7 series than before the introduction of the vaccine.

Summary

Since its licensure in 2000, inclusion of PCV7 in the childhood vaccine schedule has had a dramatic effect on the incidence of invasive pneumococcal disease in young children, with a milder but statistically significant decrease in invasive disease in their adult contacts. The effect on non-invasive pneumococcal disease in children has been less marked, but may improve as the proportion of completely immunized children expands, and the benefits of herd immunity are more fully realized. Universal immunization with PCV7 also is beginning to decrease the incidence of pneumococcal disease caused by antibiotic-resistant strains. Phenomena that may erode the benefits of the PCV7 immunization program in the future, particularly serotype replacement and serotype switching, already have been identified, but their impact is not yet defined.

References

[1] Advisory Committee on Immunization Practices. Preventing pneumococcal disease among infants and young children. MMWR Morb Mort Wkly Rep 2000;49 RR-9:1–35.

[2] American Academy of Pediatrics. Policy statement: recommendations for the prevention of pneumococcal infections, including the use of pneumococcal conjugate vaccine (Prevar), pneumococcal polysaccharide vaccine, and antibiotic prophylaxis. Pediatrics 2000;106: 362–6.

[3] CDC. Notice to readers: updated recommendations on the use of pneumococcal conjugate vaccine: suspension of recommendation for third and fourth dose. MMWR Morb Mort Wkly Rep 2004;53:177–8.

[4] CDC. National, state, and urban area vaccination coverage among children aged 19–35 months—United States, 2003. MMWR Morb Mort Wkly Rep 2004;53:658–61.

[5] Black S, Shinefield H, Baxter R, et al. Postlicensure surveillance for pneumococcal invasive disease after use of heptavalent pneumococcal conjugate vaccine in Northern California Kaiser Permanente. Pediatr Infect Dis J 2004;23:485–9.

[6] Joloba ML, Windau A, Bajaksouzian S, Appelbaum PC, Hausdorff WP, Jacobs MR. Pneumococcal conjugate vaccine serotypes of *Streptococcus pneumoniae* isolates and the antimicrobial susceptibility of such isolates in children with otitis media. Clin Infect Dis 2001;33:1489–94.

[7] Feikin DR, Klugman KP. Historical changes in pneumococcal serogroup distribution: implications for the era of pneumococcal conjugate vaccines. Clin Infect Dis 2002;35:547–55.

[8] Kayhty H, Ahman H, Ronnberg PR, Tillikainen R, Eskola J. Pneumococcal polysaccharide-meningococcal outer membrane protein complex conjugate vaccine is immunogenic in infants and children. J Infect Dis 1995;172:1273–8.

[9] Rennels MB, Edwards KM, Keyserling HL, et al. Safety and immunogenicity of heptavalent pneumococcal vaccine conjugated to CRM197 in United States infants. Pediatrics 1998;101: 604–11.

[10] Ahman H, Kayhty H, Vuorela A, Leroy O, Eskola J. Dose dependency of antibody response in infants and children to pneumococcal polysaccharides conjugated to tetanus toxoid. Vaccine 1999;17:2726–32.

[11] Black S, Shinefield H, Fireman B, et al. Efficacy, safety and immunogenicity of heptavalent pneumococcal conjugate vaccine in children. Northern California Kaiser Permanente Vaccine Study Center Group. Pediatr Infect Dis J 2000;19:187–95.

[12] Shinefield HR, Black S, Ray P, et al. Safety and immunogenicity of heptavalent pneumococcal CRM197 conjugate vaccine in infants and toddlers. Pediatr Infect Dis J 1999;18:757–63.

[13] Ahman H, Kayhty H, Lehtonen H, Leroy O, Froeschle J, Eskola J. *Streptococcus pneumoniae* capsular polysaccharide-diphtheria toxoid conjugate vaccine is immunogenic in early infancy and able to induce immunologic memory. Pediatr Infect Dis J 1998;17:211–6.

[14] Stack AM, Malley R, Thompson CM, Kobzik L, Siber GR, Saladino RA. Minimum protective serum concentrations of pneumococcal anti-capsular antibodies in infant rats. J Infect Dis 1998;177:986–90.
[15] Dagan R, Melamed R, Muallem M, et al. Reduction of nasopharyngeal carriage of pneumococci during the second year of life by a heptavalent conjugate pneumococcal vaccine. J Infect Dis 1996;174:1271–8.
[16] Dagan R, Givon-Lavi N, Zamir O, et al. Reduction of nasopharyngeal carriage of *Streptococcus pneumoniae* after administration of a 9-valent pneumococcal conjugate vaccine to toddlers attending day care centers. J Infect Dis 2002;185:927–36.
[17] Dagan R, Muallem M, Melamed R, Leroy O, Yagupsky P. Reduction of pneumococcal nasopharyngeal carriage in early infancy after immunization with tetravalent pneumococcal vaccines conjugated to either tetanus toxoid or diphtheria toxoid. Pediatr Infect Dis J 1997; 16:1060–4.
[18] Mbelle N, Huebner RE, Wasas AD, Kimura A, Chang I, Klugman KP. Immunogenicity and impact on nasopharyngeal carriage of a nonavalent pneumococcal conjugate vaccine. J Infect Dis 1999;180:1171–6.
[19] Obaro SK, Adegbola RA, Banya WA, Greenwood BM. Carriage of pneumococci after pneumococcal vaccination. Lancet 1996;348:271–2.
[20] Finkelstein JA, Huang SS, Daniel J, et al. Antibiotic-resistant *Streptococcus pneumoniae* in the heptavalent pneumococcal conjugate vaccine era: predictors of carriage in a multi-community sample. Pediatrics 2003;112:862–9.
[21] Black SB, Shinefield HR, Hansen J, Elvin L, Laufer D, Malinoski F. Postlicensure evaluation of the effectiveness of seven valent pneumococcal conjugate vaccine. Pediatr Infect Dis J 2001;20:1105–7.
[22] Flannery B, Schrag S, Bennett NM, et al. Impact of childhood vaccination on racial disparities in invasive *Streptococcus pneumoniae* infections. JAMA 2004;291:2197–203.
[23] Klugman KP, Madhi SA, Huebner RE, Kohberger R, Mbelle N, Pierce N. A trial of a 9-valent pneumococcal conjugate vaccine in children with and those without HIV infection. N Engl J Med 2003;349:1341–8.
[24] Whitney CG, Farley MM, Hadler J, et al. Decline in invasive pneumococcal disease after the introduction of protein-polysaccharide conjugate vaccine. N Engl J Med 2003;348:1737–46.
[25] Shafinoori S, Ginocchio CC, Greenberg AJ, Yeoman E, Cheddie M, Rubin LG. Impact of pneumococcal conjugate vaccine and the severity of winter influenza-like illnesses on invasive pneumococcal infections in children and adults. Pediatr Infect Dis J 2005;24:10–6.
[26] Kaplan SL, Mason EO Jr, Wald ER, et al. Decrease of invasive pneumococcal infections in children among 8 children's hospitals in the United States after the introduction of the 7-valent pneumococcal conjugate vaccine. Pediatrics 2004;113:443–9.
[27] Stephens DS, Zughaier SM, Whitney CG, et al. Incidence of macrolide resistance in *Streptococcus pneumoniae* after introduction of the pneumococcal conjugate vaccine: population-based assessment. Lancet 2005;365:855–63.
[28] Hsu K, Pelton S, Karumuri S, Heisey-Grove D, Klein J. Population-based surveillance for childhood invasive pneumococcal disease in the era of conjugate vaccine. Pediatr Infect Dis J 2005;24:17–23.
[29] Lin PL, Michaels MG, Janosky J, Ortenzo M, Wald ER, Mason EO Jr. Incidence of invasive pneumococcal disease in children 3 to 36 months of age at a tertiary care pediatric center 2 years after licensure of the pneumococcal conjugate vaccine. Pediatrics 2003;111:896–9.
[30] French N, Nakiyingi J, Carpenter LM, et al. 23-valent pneumococcal polysaccharide vaccine in HIV-1-infected Ugandan adults: double-blind, randomised and placebo controlled trial. Lancet 2000;355:2106–11.
[31] Black SB, Shinefield HR, Ling S, et al. Effectiveness of heptavalent pneumococcal conjugate vaccine in children younger than five years of age for prevention of pneumonia. Pediatr Infect Dis J 2002;21:810–5.

[32] Butler JC, Breiman RF, Lipman HB, Hofmann J, Facklam RR. Serotype distribution of *Streptococcus pneumoniae* infections among preschool children in the United States, 1978–1994: implications for development of a conjugate vaccine. J Infect Dis 1995;171:885–9.
[33] Eskola J, Kilpi T, Palmu A, et al. Efficacy of a pneumococcal conjugate vaccine against acute otitis media. N Engl J Med 2001;344:403–9.
[34] Fireman B, Black SB, Shinefield HR, Lee J, Lewis E, Ray P. Impact of the pneumococcal conjugate vaccine on otitis media. Pediatr Infect Dis J 2003;22:10–6.
[35] Veenhoven R, Bogaert D, Uiterwaal C, et al. Effect of conjugate pneumococcal vaccine followed by polysaccharide pneumococcal vaccine on recurrent acute otitis media: a randomised study. Lancet 2003;361:2189–95.
[36] Teele DW, Klein JO, Rosner B. Epidemiology of otitis media during the first seven years of life in children in greater Boston: a prospective, cohort study. J Infect Dis 1989;160:83–94.
[37] Berman S. Otitis media in children. N Engl J Med 1995;332:1560–5.
[38] McCaig LF, Besser RE, Hughes JM. Trends in antimicrobial prescribing rates for children and adolescents. JAMA 2002;287:3096–102.
[39] Zhou F, Bisgard KM, Yusuf HR, Deuson RR, Bath SK, Murphy TV. Impact of universal *Haemophilus influenzae* type b vaccination starting at 2 months of age in the United States: an economic analysis. Pediatrics 2002;110:653–61.
[40] Lieu TA, Ray GT, Black SB, et al. Projected cost-effectiveness of pneumococcal conjugate vaccination of healthy infants and young children. JAMA 2000;283:1460–8.
[41] CDC. Estimated vaccination coverage with 3 + doses of pneumococcal conjugate vaccine among children 19–35 months of age by race/ethnicity and by state and immunization action plan area. US National Immunization Survey Q1/2002–Q4/2002. Available at: http://www.cdc.gov/nip/coverage/NIS/02/tab29a_3pcv_race_iap.xls. Accessed April 11, 2005.
[42] Whitney CG, Farley MM, Hadler J, et al. Increasing prevalence of multidrug-resistant *Streptococcus pneumoniae* in the United States. N Engl J Med 2000;343:1917–24.
[43] Dagan R, Fraser D. Conjugate pneumococcal vaccine and antibiotic-resistant *Streptococcus pneumoniae*: herd immunity and reduction of otitis morbidity. Pediatr Infect Dis J 2000;19:S79–87.
[44] Casey JR, Pichichero ME. Changes in frequency and pathogens causing acute otitis media in 1995–2003. Pediatr Infect Dis J 2004;23:824–8.
[45] Beall B, McEllistrem MC, Gertz RE Jr, et al. Emergence of a novel penicillin-nonsusceptible, invasive serotype 35B clone of *Streptococcus pneumoniae* within the United States. J Infect Dis 2002;186:118–22.
[46] Porat N, Barkai G, Jacobs MR, Trefler R, Dagan R. Four antibiotic-resistant *Streptococcus pneumoniae* clones unrelated to the pneumococcal conjugate vaccine serotypes, including 2 new serotypes, causing acute otitis media in southern Israel. J Infect Dis 2004;189:385–92.
[47] Reichler MR, Allphin AA, Breiman RF, et al. The spread of multiply resistant *Streptococcus pneumoniae* at a day care center in Ohio. J Infect Dis 1992;166:1346–53.
[48] Dagan R, Melamed R, Muallem M, Piglansky L, Yagupsky P. Nasopharyngeal colonization in southern Israel with antibiotic-resistant pneumococci during the first 2 years of life: relation to serotypes likely to be included in pneumococcal conjugate vaccines. J Infect Dis 1996;174:1352–5.
[49] Gwaltney JM Jr, Sande MA, Austrian R, Hendley JO. Spread of *Streptococcus pneumoniae* in families: II. relation of transfer of *S. pneumoniae* to incidence of colds and serum antibody. J Infect Dis 1975;132:62–8.
[50] Shimada J, Yamanaka N, Hotomi M, et al. Household transmission of *Streptococcus pneumoniae* among siblings with acute otitis media. J Clin Microbiol 2002;40:1851–3.
[51] Givon-Lavi N, Fraser D, Porat N, Dagan R. Spread of *Streptococcus pneumoniae* and antibiotic-resistant *S. pneumoniae* from day-care center attendees to their younger siblings. J Infect Dis 2002;186:1608–14.

[52] Takala AK, Eskola J, Leinonen M, et al. Reduction of oropharyngeal carriage of *Haemophilus influenzae* type b (Hib) in children immunized with an Hib conjugate vaccine. J Infect Dis 1991;164:982–6.
[53] Murphy TV, Pastor P, Medley F, Osterholm MT, Granoff DM. Decreased *Haemophilus* colonization in children vaccinated with *Haemophilus influenzae* type b conjugate vaccine. J Pediatr 1993;122:517–23.
[54] Block SL, Hedrick JA, Hartrison CJ. Widespread use of conjugated pneumococcal vaccine significantly reduces rates of AOM and antibiotic usage [Abstract 1135]. Presented at Pediatric Academic Societies. San Francisco, 2004.
[55] Leibovitz E, Raiz S, Piglansky L, et al. Resistance pattern of middle ear fluid isolates in acute otitis media recently treated with antibiotics. Pediatr Infect Dis J 1998;17:463–9.
[56] Lopez B, Cima MD, Vazquez F, et al. Epidemiological study of *Streptococcus pneumoniae* carriers in healthy primary-school children. Eur J Clin Microbiol Infect Dis 1999;18:771–6.
[57] del Castillo F, Baquero-Artigao F, Garcia-Perea A. Influence of recent antibiotic therapy on antimicrobial resistance of *Streptococcus pneumoniae* in children with acute otitis media in Spain. Pediatr Infect Dis J 1998;17:94–7.
[58] Dagan R, Sikuler-Cohen M, Zamir O, Janco J, Givon-Lavi N, Fraser D. Effect of a conjugate pneumococcal vaccine on the occurrence of respiratory infections and antibiotic use in day-care center attendees. Pediatr Infect Dis J 2001;20:951–8.
[59] Block SL, Hedrick J, Harrison CJ, et al. Community-wide vaccination with the heptavalent pneumococcal conjugate significantly alters the microbiology of acute otitis media. Pediatr Infect Dis J 2004;23:829–33.
[60] Regev-Yochay G, Dagan R, Raz M, et al. Association between carriage of *Streptococcus pneumoniae* and *Staphylococcus aureus* in children. JAMA 2004;292:716–20.
[61] Nesin M, Ramirez M, Tomasz A. Capsular transformation of a multidrug-resistant *Streptococcus pneumoniae* in vivo. J Infect Dis 1998;177:707–13.
[62] Nilsson P, Laurell MH. Carriage of penicillin-resistant *Streptococcus pneumoniae* by children in day-care centers during an intervention program in Malmo, Sweden. Pediatr Infect Dis J 2001;20:1144–9.
[63] Barnes DM, Whittier S, Gilligan PH, Soares S, Tomasz A, Henderson FW. Transmission of multidrug-resistant serotype 23F *Streptococcus pneumoniae* in group day care: evidence suggesting capsular transformation of the resistant strain in vivo. J Infect Dis 1995;171:890–6.
[64] Gherardi G, Whitney CG, Facklam RR, Beall B. Major related sets of antibiotic-resistant pneumococci in the United States as determined by pulsed-field gel electrophoresis and pbp1a-pbp2b-pbp2x-dhf restriction profiles. J Infect Dis 2000;181:216–29.
[65] Coffey TJ, Enright MC, Daniels M, et al. Recombinational exchanges at the capsular polysaccharide biosynthetic locus lead to frequent serotype changes among natural isolates of *Streptococcus pneumoniae*. Mol Microbiol 1998;27:73–83.
[66] Coffey TJ, Dowson CG, Daniels M, et al. Horizontal transfer of multiple penicillin-binding protein genes, and capsular biosynthetic genes, in natural populations of *Streptococcus pneumoniae*. Mol Microbiol 1991;5:2255–60.
[67] Kelly T, Dillard JP, Yother J. Effect of genetic switching of capsular type on virulence of *Streptococcus pneumoniae*. Infect Immun 1994;62:1813–9.
[68] McEllistrem MC, Adams J, Mason EO, Wald ER. Epidemiology of acute otitis media caused by *Streptococcus pneumoniae* before and after licensure of the 7-valent pneumococcal protein conjugate vaccine. J Infect Dis 2003;188:1679–84.
[69] Klein JO. Management of the febrile child without a focus of infection in the era of universal pneumococcal immunization. Pediatr Infect Dis J 2002;21:584–8.
[70] Kuppermann N. The evaluation of young febrile children for occult bacteremia: time to reevaluate our approach? Arch Pediatr Adolesc Med 2002;156:855–7.
[71] Jaffe DM, Tanz RR, Davis AT, Henretig F, Fleisher G. Antibiotic administration to treat possible occult bacteremia in febrile children. N Engl J Med 1987;317:1175–80.

[72] McGowan JE Jr, Bratton L, Klein JO, Finland M. Bacteremia in febrile children seen in a "walk-in" pediatric clinic. N Engl J Med 1973;288:1309–12.
[73] Baraff LJ, Bass JW, Fleisher GR, et al. Practice guideline for the management of infants and children 0 to 36 months of age with fever without source. Agency for Health Care Policy and Research. Ann Emerg Med 1993;22:1198–210.
[74] Alpern ER, Alessandrini EA, Bell LM, Shaw KN, McGowan KL. Occult bacteremia from a pediatric emergency department: current prevalence, time to detection, and outcome. Pediatrics 2000;106:505–11.
[75] Lee GM, Harper MB. Risk of bacteremia for febrile young children in the post-*Haemophilus influenzae* type b era. Arch Pediatr Adolesc Med 1998;152:624–8.
[76] Stoll ML, Rubin LG. Incidence of occult bacteremia among highly febrile young children in the era of the pneumococcal conjugate vaccine: a study from a Children's Hospital Emergency Department and Urgent Care Center. Arch Pediatr Adolesc Med 2004;158: 671–5.
[77] Yamamoto LG. Revising the decision analysis for febrile children at risk for occult bacteremia in a future era of widespread pneumococcal immunization. Clin Pediatr (Phila) 2001;40:583–94.
[78] Lee GM, Fleisher GR, Harper MB. Management of febrile children in the age of the conjugate pneumococcal vaccine: a cost-effectiveness analysis. Pediatrics 2001;108:835–44.
[79] Lee KC, Finkelstein JA, Miroshnik IL, et al. Pediatricians' self-reported clinical practices and adherence to national immunization guidelines after the introduction of pneumococcal conjugate vaccine. Arch Pediatr Adolesc Med 2004;158:695–701.

ELSEVIER
SAUNDERS

Infect Dis Clin N Am 19 (2005) 647–665

INFECTIOUS
DISEASE CLINICS
OF NORTH AMERICA

Infection Control, Hospital Epidemiology, and Patient Safety

Susan E. Coffin, MD, MPH[a,c],
Theoklis E. Zaoutis, MD, MSCE[a,b,c,*]

[a] *Department of Pediatrics, University of Pennsylvania School of Medicine, Philadelphia, PA 19104, USA*
[b] *Center for Clinical Epidemiology and Biostatistics, University of Pennsylvania School of Medicine, Philadelphia, PA 19104, USA*
[c] *Division of Infectious Diseases, Children's Hospital of Philadelphia, 34th and Civic Center Boulevard, Philadelphia, PA 19104, USA*

Health care-acquired infections a major threat to the safety of hospitalized children

Nosocomial infections are the most common adverse event experienced by hospitalized patients; more recent data suggest that 10% of patients develop a nosocomial infection during admission to an acute care hospital [1]. Hospital-acquired infections (HAI) increase morbidity, extend hospital stays, and increase hospital charges [2]. They also are associated with substantial increases in in-hospital mortality [3].

Analysis of discharge data from more than 5 million pediatric hospitalizations revealed that "postoperative sepsis" and "infection as a result of medical care" were common events among hospitalized children [3], with consequences similar to the consequences seen in adults. Children who developed one a nosocomial infection were found to have increased length of hospital stay, direct health care costs, and in-hospital mortality. These findings persisted even after adjustment for patient and hospital characteristics (Table 1). The risk of HAI is significant and the consequences are great. All members of a health care team need to be aware of all that they can do to prevent patients from acquiring a nosocomial infection.

* Corresponding author. Division of Infectious Diseases, Children's Hospital of Philadelphia, 34th and Civic Center Boulevard, Philadelphia, PA 19104, USA.
E-mail address: zaoutis@email.chop.edu (T.E. Zaoutis).

0891-5520/05/$ - see front matter
doi:10.1016/j.idc.2005.05.002 **id.theclinics.com**

Table 1
Impact of nosocomial infections in hospitalized children

	Mean increase length of hospital stay (days)	Mean increase hospital charges (US dollars)	Mean increase in-hospital mortality (odds ratio)
Infection as a result of medical care	30	121,010	2.2
Postoperative sepsis	26	117,815	11

Data from Miller MR, Elixhauser A, Zhan C. Patient safety events during pediatric hospitalizations. Pediatrics 2003;111:1358–66.

Similarities between classic epidemiology and new quality improvement techniques

Although often compartmentalized, infection control and hospital epidemiology should be well integrated into a hospital's quality improvement and patient safety activities [4–7]. In addition to shared goals—improved patient outcomes—the work processes used by these groups are similar. Although the quality improvement movement has adopted distinctive language to describe its analytic approaches, many quality improvement activities are rooted in classic epidemiology. Infection control professionals and quality improvement managers rely on active surveillance to gather data about patient outcomes and process measures. Members of an infection control department monitor outcomes such as the rates of specific health care–associated infections and process measures such as compliance with hand hygiene guidelines or timing of perioperative antibiotics. Similarly, quality improvement teams measure outcomes such as medication errors and process measures such as use of appropriate patient identification strategies. Through the presentation of data collected from observations and active surveillance to clinicians caring for at-risk patients, both groups work to motivate and sustain changes in medical practice. Patient safety officers and infection control professionals target systematic barriers to optimal patient care and frequently rely on process analysis (often referred to as root-cause analysis by quality professionals) to identify unrecognized barriers to optimal care. Interviews and direct observations commonly are employed by both groups to perform these analyses. Finally, basic techniques of outbreak investigation often are adopted when a patient safety team recognizes a new threat to patient safety, such as medication errors [8]. Typically a successful investigation by either infection control professionals or quality improvement managers culminates in the introduction of one or more interventions coupled with ongoing surveillance to evaluate the impact.

Using reference data

The National Nosocomial Infections Surveillance (NNIS) system of the Centers for Disease Control and Prevention (CDC) provides rates of HAI in pediatric patients [9] and compiles data from pediatric institutions that voluntarily report HAI that occur in neonatal intensive care unit (NICU) or pediatric intensive care unit (PICU) patients. The availability of such aggregated data has provided much sought-after reference rates for individual facilities. More recently, other organizations have begun to create voluntary reporting systems to collect and aggregate a variety of administrative and patient safety information to assist participating hospitals in quality improvement activities. There are important caveats, however, that limit the utility of such reference data. First, there is often considerable variability between individual hospitals that choose to participate within a single benchmark system. NNIS compiles data on bloodstream infections that occur in NICU patients. Institutions that contribute data range from level-two community NICU to level-three NICU within a freestanding children's hospital. So far, few benchmarking systems provide the tools needed to compare rates at peer institutions or to adjust for case mix. Second, the resources available to individual hospitals that participate in benchmarking groups often vary. As previously shown, the method used to collect data [10] and the ratio between patient beds and infection control professionals significantly influence the quality of surveillance data. Finally, standard definitions of specific HAI have been put forth by the NNIS and widely adopted by hospital departments of infection control. These definitions are designed to facilitate surveillance, however, and at times may be at odds with clinically relevant definitions of infection. In addition, interpretation of standard definitions can vary [11].

In an attempt to define better HAI rates in US children's hospitals, the CDC established the Pediatric Prevention Network (PPN) in collaboration with the National Association of Children's Hospitals and Related Institutions. The PPN was established to determine HAI rates and to develop and test infection prevention interventions in children's hospitals. Despite concerns about the quality of pediatric HAI data compiled by NNIS, the PPN found median rates of HAI from PPN hospitals' NICU and PICU were comparable to NNIS rates.

Public reporting of health care–associated infections

Accountability and transparency are two qualities that US patients increasingly have demanded of their health care system [12]. In addition, public and private insurers increasingly request evidence that the care rendered at an individual institution is cost-efficient. In response to these concerns, five states have instituted regulations that require acute care hospitals to report some or all HAI. At present, the reporting requirements vary greatly. In some states, currently reported data are unlikely to be meaningful because of variations in resources available and methods used to conduct surveillance. As additional states introduce similar legislation, however, leaders in hospital epidemiology will have an opportunity to guide the development of these programs and perhaps establish a national system to provide patients with understandable and accurate data about the risk of HAI in hospitals in their community.

Transmission of pathogens within a pediatric health care setting

To prevent nosocomial infections, health care providers must understand how organisms are transmitted between persons, how and when colonizing organisms (often referred to as *commensal organisms*) can become pathogenic, and how host and environmental factors modify the risk of nosocomial infection. Three basic mechanisms explain how most microorganisms are transmitted from one person to another. The routes of transmission of common pediatric organisms are summarized in Table 2.

Contact transmission

Contact is the most common route by which bacteria and viruses are spread among patients and health care workers. Viruses (e.g., respiratory

Table 2
Summary of expanded precautions for selected pathogens

Organism	Precautions[a]	Comments
Virus		
Adenovirus	C + D	Contact only for patients with isolated conjunctivitis or gastroenteritis
Enterovirus	C	
Influenza virus	D	
Parainfluenza virus	C	
Respiratory syncytial virus	C	
Rotavirus	C	
Rubeola virus (measles)	AII	
Varicella virus	C + AII	Continue until all lesions are crusted. C only needed for immunocompetent patients with zoster
Bacteria		
Antibiotic-resistant organisms[b]	C	
Bordetella pertussis	D	Continue for 5 d after initiation of appropriate therapy
Clostridium difficile	C	
Mycobacterium tuberculosis	AII	AII required only for suspected cavitary, laryngeal, or miliary disease
Mycoplasma pneumoniae	D	
Neisseria meningitidis	D	Continue for 24 h after initiation of appropriate therapy

[a] Categories of precautions: C, contact; D, droplet; AII, airborne infection isolation.
[b] Including methicillin-resistant *Staphylococcus aureus,* vancomycin-resistant *Enterococcus,* pan-resistant gram-negative rods.

syncytial virus [RSV]) and bacteria (e.g., methicillin-resistant *Staphylococcus aureus* [MRSA]) typically are spread directly between patients. For hospitalized children, contact within a hospital playroom between infected (or colonized) and susceptible children has been a frequent mode of transmission [13]. Indirect contact or fomite transmission is another common way that organisms, especially those capable of surviving for long periods on inanimate objects, can spread within the hospital [14].

Droplet transmission

Respiratory droplets are responsible for the transmission of many common pediatric pathogens, including influenza and parainfluenza viruses. Large respiratory droplets that contain viral particles are expelled from the nose and mouth during coughing, sneezing, and talking. These droplets can travel 3 to 6 feet in the air before settling. Face-to-face contact with an infected individual provides opportunity for transmission of many viral pathogens in the absence of direct physical contact.

Airborne transmission

Some organisms can become airborne and travel significant distances from their point of origin. Organisms such as *Mycobacterium tuberculosis*, varicella virus, and measles virus can survive desiccation and exist as droplet nuclei, minute particles that can remain suspended in air for long periods. The outbreak potential for these organisms is great [15]. Despite the relatively rapid adoption of the varicella vaccine, children with primary varicella infection remain a frequent source of occupational and nosocomial exposures in pediatric facilities [16].

Prevention of health care–acquired infections: general principles

Hand hygiene and standard precautions

Hand hygiene remains the most crucial element of prevention of nosocomial infections. It also is a practice that is commonly overlooked by many individuals responsible for providing hands-on patient care [17]. Health care workers are one of the most frequent sources of transmission of infection between patients. Hands should be washed with soap and water before and after eating, after using the bathroom, and when visibly soiled. At all other times, health care providers should use alcohol-based hand rubs [17]. Compared with soap and water, alcohol hand rubs are more effective at reducing microbial colonization of hands [18].

In addition to performing hand hygiene before and after every patient contact, all health care workers should observe standard precautions with every patient. Standard precautions are transmission-based precautions designed to protect health care workers from exposure to any known or unknown pathogens that might be transmitted by contact with blood or body fluids. Crucial elements of standard precautions include (1) hand hygiene; (2) gloves when touching blood, body fluids, mucous membranes, or nonintact skin; and (3) mask, gown, and eye protection during procedures that might result in sprays of blood or body fluids.

The pediatric environment of care also can pose unique infection control challenges. First, size matters. The small size of many pediatric patients increases the possibility of autocontamination. For an infant who has undergone surgical repair of congenital heart diseases, a small distance often separates a heavily colonized endotracheal tube and the proximal margin of a fresh mediastinal incision. Second, novel technologies designed to improve the care of small patients can bring with them novel hazards. The development of isolettes revolutionized the care of premature infants. The high humidity that they were designed to provide patients with immature skin also can serve as a breeding ground for opportunistic pathogens, however, such as *Serratia* [19]. In addition, the confined space within an isolette poses significant challenges to clinicians who must maintain an awareness of clean and dirty zones within the small area [20]. Many pediatric facilities have responded to the developmental needs of hospitalized children by providing playrooms on hospital wards. Numerous outbreaks have been traced to direct and indirect contact between infected or colonized and susceptible patients [21]. Achieving the appropriate balance between satisfying the developmental needs of sick children and preventing transmission of critical pathogens remains a serious challenge for most pediatric hospital epidemiologists.

Expanded precautions and the use of personal protective equipment

In addition to standard precautions, expanded precautions markedly reduce the risk of transmission of many common agents of health care–acquired infections [22]. Because many community-acquired pediatric pathogens are spread easily on inpatient units that care for children, the use of expanded precautions is especially important for facilities and units that care for children. Expanded precautions are designed to inhibit the likely modes of transmission of specific microorganisms (see earlier) and include (1) contact, (2) droplet, and (3) airborne infection isolation. Some infections can be spread in multiple ways, necessitating the simultaneous use of multiple precautionary strategies (e.g., contact and airborne infection isolation for children hospitalized with primary varicella infection).

Health care workers must understand the need for and appropriate use of personal protective equipment that forms the core of transmission-based precautions. There is consensus that barrier precautions should be used to reduce the transmission of MRSA in hospitals [23,24]. In an investigation that included weekly cultures of patients and personnel, molecular typing of isolates, and decolonization of some patients, investigators found that when patients colonized or infected with MRSA were not cared for under contact precautions, MRSA was spread to other patients at a rate of 0.14 transmissions per day [25]. In contrast, when health care workers caring for patients with MRSA used gowns and gloves, the rate of MRSA transmission to other patients was 0.009 transmissions per day. The risk of transmission was reduced nearly 16-fold when MRSA patients were cared for using contact precautions [25].

Epidemiology of pediatric health care–acquired infections

The epidemiology of HAI has been well described in adult populations [26–29]; however, such data cannot be extrapolated to pediatric patients. As is the case with other clinical situations, children are not simply little adults. The differences between adult and pediatric populations include age; birth weight considerations; and distribution of nosocomial infections by site, pathogen, and device use. Within the pediatric population, there are differences between neonates and older children. Most studies of HAI in children have focused on the populations located in the NICU and the PICU [30–36]. These units in children's hospitals provide highly specialized care for many of the most critically ill infants and children, the patient populations at greatest risk for HAI.

Advances in neonatology have improved the survival of very-low-birth-weight infants (infants <1500 g) and have resulted in a unique population of infants at high risk for HAI [37]. These infants require invasive monitoring and supportive care and are immunologically immature secondary to prematurity. Premature neonates lack transplacentally acquired maternal antibodies and have defects in complement and neutrophil function and cellular immunity [38,39]. Newborns begin life without normal bacterial flora to provide colonization resistance against nosocomially acquired pathogens. In addition to the common routes of entry of nosocomial pathogens seen in other patient populations (e.g., respiratory tract and gastrointestinal tract), premature neonates have fragile skin that is easily traumatized, resulting in bacterial invasion by colonizing flora [38,39].

Older children who are critically or chronically ill and are cared for in a PICU also possess characteristics that distinguish them from adults regarding their risk for HAI [2,36]. On the one hand, relatively few children compared with adults have chronic or degenerative disorders; most children treated in a PICU lack comorbidities that are independently associated with an increased risk of HAI [40]. On the other hand, fewer technologies designed to reduce the risk of HAI are available to pediatric patients. Antibiotic-impregnated central venous catheters have been neither approved by the Food and Drug Administration nor endorsed by the CDC or American Academy of Pediatrics for use in children [41]. The patient populations in a PICU are heterogeneous. In contrast to adult intensive care units (ICUs), most hospitals that care for critically ill children do not segregate medical and surgical patients [42]. In addition, many general hospitals lack a dedicated PICU and pediatric intensivists.

More recent reports have shown that bloodstream infections (BSI), pneumonia, and urinary tract infections (UTI) account for almost two thirds of HAI in PICU patients [32]. The distribution of HAI among children is shown in Table 3. In contrast to critically ill adult patients [43], BSI are the most common nosocomial infection experienced by pediatric patients. This difference may reflect the lower rate of urinary catheter use in pediatric compared with adult patients (Table 4) [32,43,44].

Infections related to medical devices

Most data on the risk factors for health care–acquired infections are derived from adult populations. A prospective cohort study of PICU patients identified operative status, a high PRISM (pediatric risk of mortality) score, device use ratio, antimicrobial therapy, parenteral nutrition, and length of stay before onset of infection as independent risk factors for a health care–acquired infection [33]. In neonates, birth weight has been inversely associated with the risk of nosocomial infection [34].

In all age groups, medical devices greatly increase the risk of nosocomial infection. Central venous catheters, urinary catheters, and endotracheal tubes all provide portals of entry that permit organisms to migrate from the skin and mucous membranes to sterile body sites. Implantable devices also can disrupt host defenses and provide a site sequestered from the surveillance of the immune system where bacteria can flourish. The strict adherence to aseptic technique when placing or manipulating a medical device is crucial to prevent device-related infections. Additional strategies

Table 3
Types of hospital-acquired infections reported from patients cared for in pediatric intensive care units

Infection	≤2 mo (%)	>2 mo to ≤5 y (%)	>5 y to ≤12 y (%)	>12 y (%)
Bloodstream	34	28	21	25
Pneumonia	18	20	26	21
Urinary tract	12	14	17	22
Surgical site infection	10	6	7	6
Other[a]	26	32	29	26

[a] Includes eye, ear, nose, and throat infection; gastrointestinal infection; skin and soft tissue infection; cardiovascular infection; and others.

Data from Richards MJ, Edwards JR, Culver DH, Gaynes RP. Nosocomial infections in pediatric intensive care units in the United States. National Nosocomial Infections Surveillance System. Pediatrics 1999;103:e39.

Table 4
Pooled means of device-associated infection rates by type of intensive care unit, January 2002 through June 2004

Type of ICU	CLABSI[a]	VAP[b]	UTI[c]
NICU			
≤1000 g[d]	9.1	3.5	NA
1001–1500 g	5.4	2.4	NA
1501–2500 g	4.1	1.9	NA
>2500 g	3.5	1.4	NA
Pediatric ICU	6.6	2.9	4
Adult ICUs			
Coronary	3.5	4.4	4.5
Medical	5	4.9	5.1
Medical/surgical	4	5.4	3.9
Surgical	4.6	9.3	4.4
Burn	7	12	6.7

[a] Central line–associated bloodstream infection rate/1000 central line days.
[b] Ventilator-associated pneumonia rate/1000 ventilator days.
[c] Urinary catheter–associated urinary tract infection rate/1000 urinary catheter days.
[d] Birth weight.
Data from cumulative data collected through National Nosocomial Infection Surveillance.

are outlined next that have been proven to reduce the risk of HAI in patients who require advanced medical technologies.

Central venous catheters

BSI are not only among the most common, but also among the most expensive health care–acquired infections experienced by hospitalized children. Elward et al [2] estimated that the attributable cost of catheter-related BSI in PICU patients was approximately $39,000. Although the risk of infection is greatest among patients with nontunneled central venous catheters, all vascular catheters, including peripheral intravenous catheters, are associated with an increased risk of infection [45]. Catheter-associated infections include localized infections at the site of catheter entry, phlebitis, and BSI. Practices associated with a reduced risk of catheter-associated infections include (1) use of maximal sterile barriers during catheter placement, (2) use of chlorhexidine/isopropyl alcohol solution to prepare the skin before placement or during routine care of the catheter, (3) prompt removal of catheters as soon as they are no longer required, and (4) strict adherence to appropriate hand hygiene practices [41]. In studies performed in adult ICUs, antiseptic-impregnated catheters have been associated with reduced rates of central line–associated BSI [46]. Although these guidelines generally pertain to children and adults, the prevention of pediatric catheter-associated infections has been hampered by limited access to new materials developed to prevent catheter-associated BSI. A solution of chlorhexidine/isopropyl alcohol for skin antisepsis has not been approved for use in infants younger than 2 months old. Similarly an adhesive dressing impregnated with chlorhexidine has been licensed for use only in patients older than 12 years of age. Finally, antibiotic-impregnated catheters have not been studied adequately in children [47]. Critically and chronically ill children do not benefit fully from the advances in care available to adult patients.

The microbiology of nosocomial BSI in some pediatric populations differs from that commonly reported for adult patients. Coagulase-negative staphylococci (CONS) account for approximately 40% of the pathogens identified in children with nosocomial BSI; in neonates, CONS account for an even greater percentage of isolates (50%) [34,36,48,49]. Gram-negative aerobic bacilli account for approximately 25% of pediatric nosocomial BSI, representing a larger proportion of the organisms isolated from critically ill children than adults.

The diagnosis of nosocomial BSI can be more difficult in children than adults. Current NNIS definitions for catheter-related BSI require that data be obtained from cultures of a catheter tip or the peripheral blood [45]. Pediatricians often are reluctant to perform peripheral blood cultures in children, however, because the procedure can be difficult and painful. In addition, removal of a catheter for diagnostic purposes is avoided because of the difficulties inherent in placing central venous catheters and the limited venous access available in children. The distinction between pathogen and contaminant is affected by age and underlying condition of the child. The role of CONS as a true pathogen in neonates has been well described, but continues to be a controversial subject [50].

Ventilator-associated pneumonia

An endotracheal tube provides an ideal portal of entry for the numerous organisms that colonize the oropharynx to migrate into the lower respiratory tract. An artificial airway also provides a substrate for the formation of biofilm and inhibits host defenses, such as the gag reflex and cilia function. The epidemiology of VAP is well described in adults, but few data exist for pediatric patients. Pediatric patients seem to be at less risk of ventilator-associated pneumonia (VAP) than adults, likely because they have fewer comorbid conditions, such as chronic heart or lung disease or immunosuppressive conditions. Pediatric intensive care physicians have embraced strategies that reduce the risk of VAP, however, including whenever possible (1) the use of noninvasive ventilation, (2) the avoidance of nasotracheal intubation, (3) the use of in-line suctioning to prevent the aspiration of pooled tracheal sections, and (4) the elevation of the head of the bed at 45° from horizontal, especially for patients receiving enteral nutrition [51]. Many, but not all, risk factors for VAP in pediatric patients are similar to the risk factors identified for adult patients; pediatric risk factors for VAP include the presence of a genetic syndrome, reintubation, neuromuscular blockade, and immunosuppression [48]. Identified risk factors for VAP in neonates include antecedent BSI and prolonged intubation [34,37].

VAP is associated with significant morbidity and mortality, particularly in neonates; the case-fatality rate for neonates with VAP has been reported to be 10%, with extremely preterm neonates having a much higher rate (27%). Among PICU patients, the rate has been reported to be approximately 6%. VAP is associated with prolonged ICU stay and prolonged hospital stay in NICU and PICU patients [48]. Mechanical ventilation, particularly when associated with nasotracheal intubation, in children also is a risk factor for sinusitis and otitis media. The use of a nasopharyngeal tube interferes with the normal drainage of the sinuses and the eustachian tube. In children, the small diameter of these structures increases the risk of obstruction and secondary infection [52,53].

As in adults, the diagnosis of VAP in children is difficult to confirm. NNIS has developed guidelines for the diagnosis of VAP in pediatric patients that are based on clinical and radiographic criteria, but the sensitivity and specificity of these criteria are poor. Advances in the diagnosis of VAP in adult patients have included the use of bronchoscopic bronchoalveolar lavage (BAL) or protected specimen brush to obtain secretions of the lower respiratory tract for quantitative bacterial culture. These invasive procedures are not used routinely in children, however, because of technical difficulties and the potential for complications. This problem is even more challenging in NICU patients because of the difficulty obtaining any specimens through the endotracheal tube other than suctioned secretions. In one of the few pediatric studies comparing different diagnostic methods in children, Gauvin et al [54] found that a quantitative culture of lower respiratory tract secretions obtained by blind, protected BAL was the most reliable diagnostic test; a bacterial index (the sum of the log of all species obtained by BAL) of greater than 5 was predictive of VAP.

In 1991, Pugin et al [55] proposed the Clinical Pulmonary Infection Score (CPIS) as a tool to identify adult ICU patients with pulmonary infection and showed good correlation between a threshold score of 6 and quantitative bacteriology of BAL samples. Subsequently, several attempts have been made to validate the CPIS in adult patients with variable results. This score subsequently was modified and evaluated as a tool to limit unnecessary antibiotic use in an adult ICU. Patients found to be at low risk for infection by the modified CPIS were managed successfully with short-course empiric antibiotic therapy [56]. Additionally, use of the modified CPIS resulted in significantly lower antimicrobial therapy costs and antibiotic resistance, without adversely affecting patient mortality and length of stay in the ICU. So far, clinical scoring systems to establish a diagnosis of bacterial pulmonary infection have not been tested in pediatric patients. The National Institutes of Health Bacteriology and Mycology Study Group is evaluating a protocol designed to derive a clinical prediction rule for bacterial pneumonia in children receiving mechanical ventilation.

Similar to adult patients with VAP, gram-negative aerobic bacilli, such as *Pseudomonas aeruginosa,* are the most common organisms recovered from

PICU patients with VAP [32,48]. NICU patients also are at risk of VAP caused by *Enterococcus* and group B *Streptococcus* [57]. In pediatric patients with VAP, viruses, such as RSV, have been recovered from the lower respiratory tract in the absence of other pathogens.

Catheter-related urinary tract infections

Similar to vascular catheters, the use of urinary catheters is associated with an increased risk of UTI. Experts estimate that catheter-associated UTI are the most common device-associated infection among hospitalized patients, although the burden of disease is likely greater in adult compared with pediatric patients. Inappropriate and prolonged use of urinary catheters has been found in 50% of patients who develop catheter-associated UTI [58,59]. Guidelines have focused on several practices that can reduce the risk of these infections [60]. First, catheters should be placed in a sterile fashion. Second, a closed system for urine collection always should be maintained. Finally, the use of urinary catheters should be minimized by prompt removal whenever possible.

Most nosocomial UTI in children are caused by gram-negative bacilli, with *E coli* as the most frequently reported isolate (19%). Fungal UTI seem to be less common in children than adults, likely due in part to differences in the prevalence of comorbid conditions and antibiotic exposure. NICU patients may be uniquely vulnerable to nosocomial UTI resulting from CONS [58,59]. Risk factors for UTI in hospitalized children include female sex and catheterization. One study of nosocomial UTI found that the median duration of catheterization before infection was 7 days [59]. In contrast to BSI, the definitions for nosocomial UTI are generally well established and easily applied to children and adults.

Epidemiology of non–device-related pediatric health care–acquired infections

Surgical site infections

As seen in adults, gram-positive cocci account for nearly half of the pathogens in children with surgical site infections [61,62]. *S aureus* is the most common organism identified after chest and cardiovascular surgery, followed by CONS. Gram-negative bacilli, including *Pseudomonas,* also are common, particularly after gastrointestinal surgery.

In pediatric studies of surgical site infections, wound class is identified as a strong predictor of infection [62]. Rates of infection by wound class are similar for adults and children. Other identified risk factors include longer duration of surgery, prolonged preoperative hospital stay, emergency surgery, longer incision length, and the presence of underlying disease. Duration of surgery was identified in the only study to use multivariate analysis to adjust for confounders. In contrast to adults, intraoperative hyperglycemia has not been found to be a major risk factor for infection in pediatric patients; this likely reflects the low prevalence of diabetes in children.

One type of pediatric surgery–associated condition warrants additional discussion. The placement of a ventriculoperitoneal shunt for management of chronic hydrocephalus is one of the most commonly performed operations in pediatric patients. The morbidity associated with shunt infections is high, and treatment includes surgery to remove the infected shunt in addition to antibiotic therapy. Current literature suggests a 5% to 10% infection rate, with half of the infections occurring within the first 2 weeks after surgery [63]. Gram-positive organisms cause most of these infections, with CONS accounting for nearly half of the infections.

Mycobacterium tuberculosis

In contrast to adults, many children infected with *M tuberculosis* are not considered contagious. Several factors explain the low rate of communicability associated with pediatric *M tuberculosis* infections [64]. First, most children infected with *M tuberculosis* have latent infection and have small numbers of organisms that are well sequestered in granulomata. Second, children with active *M tuberculosis* infection rarely have endobronchial or cavitary lesions that communicate with the lower airways. Finally, young children typically do not generate sufficient intrathoracic pressure during cough to raise *M tuberculosis* organisms into the oropharynx. Expanded precautions are not used routinely for pediatric patients with *M tuberculosis* infection. Airborne infection isolation precautions (including patient placement in a negative-pressure room and the use of high-efficiency respirator masks by health care providers) should be instituted for pediatric patients with suspected endobronchial or cavitary lesions or miliary disease. Precautions should be continued until a patient is shown to have no acid-fast organisms visible on three consecutive induced sputum specimens.

Viral pathogens

During seasonal outbreaks, common pediatric viral pathogens can pose a significant risk to hospitalized children [65]. Transmission of organisms such as RSV, influenza virus, or rotavirus is facilitated in an inpatient pediatric unit because of the relative concentration of susceptibles (ie, the patients), ongoing introduction of virus from the community (by visitors, staff, and newly admitted patients), and environmental contamination with organisms that can live for hours on fomites [66,67]. Outbreaks of rotavirus have been linked repeatedly to persistent contamination of inanimate objects despite adherence to environmental cleaning policies [68]. In addition, outbreaks have been perpetuated by unrecognized asymptomatic or subclinical infection of hospital staff or prolonged shedding of virus associated with primary infections [69–71]. Hospital outbreaks of RSV and rotavirus have been associated with insufficient staffing, suboptimal environmental cleaning, and illness among visitors and staff [65,68,69,72].

Some investigators have shown the benefits of aggressive use of viral diagnostic testing to identify and isolate cases of community-acquired viral infections (eg, RSV and rotavirus) as an important strategy to reduce the risk of nosocomial transmission of these common pediatric pathogens [69,73]. Macartney et al [73] showed that a comprehensive infection control program could reduce the frequency of nosocomial RSV infections and be cost-efficient. This model program included viral diagnostic testing, cohorting of patients and staff, use of barrier precautions, and monitoring and education and resulted in a savings of $6.00 for every dollar expended.

Multiple drug–resistant organisms

Judicious use of antibiotics

In addition to infection control practices, an important factor in the emergence of antibiotic-resistant organisms is the use of antimicrobials. Numerous studies have shown an association between the use of broad-spectrum antimicrobials and emergence of antibiotic-resistant pathogens [74–76]. Data regarding antimicrobial use in children are limited. Studies have shown that approximately 71% of patients in NICU and 43% of patients in PICU were receiving antimicrobials at the time the prevalence studies were conducted [34,77]. In both populations of critically ill children, nearly 50% of vancomycin use was empirical. Numerous studies have shown that vancomycin use in pediatric populations is excessive and not consistent with current guideline recommendations [78–80]. Analysis of data from the PPN revealed that cefazolin was the antimicrobial agent most commonly used in PICU (most patients had undergone surgery), followed by third-generation cephalosporins and vancomycin. Gentamicin was the most commonly used agent in NICU followed by ampicillin and vancomycin. In contrast, NNIS data show that third-generation cephalosporins are the most commonly used agents in PICU followed by vancomycin. Differences between these results may be explained in part by methodologic differences in measuring antimicrobial use. Measurement of antimicrobial use in NNIS does not adjust for patient weight—a factor that determines dose for virtually all antibiotics administered to pediatric patients. These data are likely to be underestimates of antimicrobial use in children.

Several interventions designed to have an impact on antimicrobial use have been evaluated in pediatric patients. A study performed in two NICU in the Netherlands reported a significant impact on the prevalence of antibiotic-resistant organisms when empirical therapy for early-onset sepsis consisted of narrow-spectrum agents versus broad-spectrum regimens [81]. In contrast, a study of ceftazidime restriction in a PICU did not result in a significant change in the overall incidence of colonization with ceftazidime-resistant gram-negative bacilli [82]. Another interesting but unproven approach to reducing antibiotic resistance is antibiotic cycling.

Toltzis et al [83] found that antibiotic cycling in a tertiary-care NICU had no detectable effect on the reservoir of resistant gram-negative bacilli. Other strategies for improving antimicrobial use have been studied, but their efficacy in reducing antibiotic resistance is unproven. These strategies include education programs, formulary restrictions, prior-approval programs, therapeutic substitution and streamlining programs, computer-assisted management programs, and combinations of the aforementioned approaches [84].

Active surveillance to identify patients colonized with multiple drug–resistant organisms

In the 1990s, multiple drug–resistant organisms emerged as a major issue for institutions that provide health care to children. In 2004, an expert panel of hospital epidemiologists recommended that hospitals consider screening all admitted patients for two multiple drug–resistant organisms that have been associated frequently with HAI, vancomycin-resistant enterococcus and MRSA [85]. Although the prevalence of vancomycin-resistant enterococcus or MRSA colonization among pediatric patients is significantly lower than that reported in most studies of adult patients [22], some pediatric hospitals have instituted targeted surveillance of defined high-risk patient populations [86]. The impact of this practice has yet to be established.

References

[1] Burke JP. Infection control—a problem for patient safety. N Engl J Med 2003;348:651–6.
[2] Elward AM, Hollenbeak CS, Warren DK, Fraser VJ. Attributable cost of nosocomial primary bloodstream infection in pediatric intensive care unit patients. Pediatrics 2005;115: 868–72.
[3] Miller MR, Elixhauser A, Zhan C. Patient safety events during pediatric hospitalizations. Pediatrics 2003;111:1358–66.
[4] Gnass SA, Barboza L, Bilicich D, et al. Prevention of central venous catheter-related bloodstream infections using non-technologic strategies. Infect Control Hosp Epidemiol 2004;25:675–7.
[5] Misset B, Timsit JF, Dumay MF, et al. A continuous quality-improvement program reduces nosocomial infection rates in the ICU. Intensive Care Med 2004;30:395–400.
[6] Scheckler WE. Healthcare epidemiology is the paradigm for patient safety. Infect Control Hosp Epidemiol 2002;23:47–51.
[7] Simonds DN, Horan TC, Kelley R, Jarvis WR. Detecting pediatric nosocomial infections: how do infection control and quality assurance personnel compare? Am J Infect Control 1997;25:202–8.
[8] Jones TF, Feler CA, Simmons BP, et al. Neurologic complications including paralysis after a medication error involving implanted intrathecal catheters. Am J Med 2002;112:31–6.
[9] Jarvis WR. Benchmarking for prevention: the Centers for Disease Control and Prevention's National Nosocomial Infections Surveillance (NNIS) system experience. Infection 2003; 31(Suppl 2):44–8.
[10] Scheckler WE, Brimhall D, Buck AS, et al. Requirements for infrastructure and essential activities of infection control and epidemiology in hospitals: a consensus panel

report. Society for Healthcare Epidemiology of America. Am J Infect Control 1998;26: 47–60.

[11] Zembower T, Tokars J, Johnson S, et al. Discrepancies in data collection for ventilator-associated pneumonia. Presented at Society for Healthcare Epidemiology of America, Los Angeles; 2005.

[12] Marshall MN, Hiscock J, Sibbald B. Attitudes to the public release of comparative information on the quality of general practice care: qualitative study. BMJ 2002;325:1278.

[13] Hall CB. Nosocomial respiratory syncytial virus infections: the "Cold War" has not ended. Clin Infect Dis 2000;31:590–6.

[14] Rogers M, Weinstock DM, Eagan J, Kiehn T, Armstrong D, Sepkowitz KA. Rotavirus outbreak on a pediatric oncology floor: possible association with toys. Am J Infect Control 2000;28:378–80.

[15] Langley JM, Hanakowski M. Variation in risk for nosocomial chickenpox after inadvertent exposure. J Hosp Infect 2000;44:224–6.

[16] Sherman E, Behrman A, Wax G, et al. Occupational and nosocomial exposures from patients with acute generalized vesicular-pustular rash illnesses. Presented at: Society for Healthcare Epidemiology of America, Los Angeles; 2005.

[17] Boyce JM, Pittet D. Guideline for hand hygiene in health-care settings. Recommendations of the Healthcare Infection Control Practices Advisory Committee and the HIPAC/SHEA/APIC/IDSA Hand Hygiene Task Force. Am J Infect Control 2002;30:S1–46.

[18] Girou E, Loyeau S, Legrand P, Oppein F, Brun-Buisson C. Efficacy of handrubbing with alcohol based solution versus standard handwashing with antiseptic soap: randomised clinical trial. BMJ 2002;325:362.

[19] Jang TN, Fung CP, Yang TL, Shen SH, Huang CS, Lee SH. Use of pulsed-field gel electrophoresis to investigate an outbreak of *Serratia marcescens* infection in a neonatal intensive care unit. J Hosp Infect 2001;48:13–9.

[20] Davenport SE. Frequency of hand washing by registered nurses caring for infants on radiant warmers and in incubators. Neonatal Netw 1992;11:21–5.

[21] Hanrahan KS, Lofgren M. Evidence-based practice: examining the risk of toys in the microenvironment of infants in the neonatal intensive care unit. Adv Neonatal Care 2004;4: 184–201.

[22] Huskins W, Goldmann D. Prevention and control of nosocomial infections in health care facilities that serve children. 5th ed. Philadelphia: Saunders; 2004.

[23] Rupp M. Control of gram-positive multidrug-resistant organisms. 1st ed. Thorofare (NJ): Slack; 2004.

[24] Cooper BS, Stone SP, Kibbler CC, et al. Isolation measures in the hospital management of methicillin resistant *Staphylococcus aureus* (MRSA): systematic review of the literature. BMJ 2004;329:533.

[25] Jernigan JA, Titus MG, Groschel DH, Getchell-White S, Farr BM. Effectiveness of contact isolation during a hospital outbreak of methicillin-resistant *Staphylococcus aureus*. Am J Epidemiol 1996;143:496–504.

[26] Bonten MJ, Kollef MH, Hall JB. Risk factors for ventilator-associated pneumonia: from epidemiology to patient management. Clin Infect Dis 2004;38:1141–9.

[27] Pittet D, Davis CS, Li N, Wenzel RP. Identifying the hospitalized patient at risk for nosocomial bloodstream infection: a population-based study. Proc Assoc Am Physicians 1997;109:58–67.

[28] Platt R, Polk BF, Murdock B, Rosner B. Risk factors for nosocomial urinary tract infection. Am J Epidemiol 1986;124:977–85.

[29] Velasco E, Thuler LC, Martins CA, Dias LM, Goncalves VM. Risk factors for bloodstream infections at a cancer center. Eur J Clin Microbiol Infect Dis 1998;17:587–90.

[30] Adams-Chapman I, Stoll BJ. Prevention of nosocomial infections in the neonatal intensive care unit. Curr Opin Pediatr 2002;14:157–64.

[31] Odetola FO, Moler FW, Dechert RE, VanDerElzen K, Chenoweth C. Nosocomial catheter-related bloodstream infections in a pediatric intensive care unit: risk and rates associated with various intravascular technologies. Pediatr Crit Care Med 2003;4:432–6.
[32] Richards MJ, Edwards JR, Culver DH, Gaynes RP. Nosocomial infections in pediatric intensive care units in the United States. National Nosocomial Infections Surveillance System. Pediatrics 1999;103:e39.
[33] Singh-Naz N, Sprague BM, Patel KM, Pollack MM. Risk factors for nosocomial infection in critically ill children: a prospective cohort study. Crit Care Med 1996;24:875–8.
[34] Sohn AH, Garrett DO, Sinkowitz-Cochran RL, et al. Prevalence of nosocomial infections in neonatal intensive care unit patients: results from the first national point-prevalence survey. J Pediatr 2001;139:821–7.
[35] Stover BH, Shulman ST, Bratcher DF, Brady MT, Levine GL, Jarvis WR. Nosocomial infection rates in US children's hospitals' neonatal and pediatric intensive care units. Am J Infect Control 2001;29:152–7.
[36] Urrea M, Pons M, Serra M, Latorre C, Palomeque A. Prospective incidence study of nosocomial infections in a pediatric intensive care unit. Pediatr Infect Dis J 2003;22:490–4.
[37] Saiman L. Risk factors for hospital-acquired infections in the neonatal intensive care unit. Semin Perinatol 2002;26:315–21.
[38] Levy O, Martin S, Eichenwald E, et al. Impaired innate immunity in the newborn: newborn neutrophils are deficient in bactericidal/permeability-increasing protein. Pediatrics 1999;104:1327–33.
[39] Lewis D, Wilson C. Developmental immunity and role of host defenses in fetal and neonatal susceptibility to infection. Philadelphia: Saunders; 2001.
[40] Crone RK. Paediatric and neonatal intensive care. Can J Anaesth 1988;35:S30–3.
[41] O'Grady NP, Alexander M, Dellinger EP, et al. Guidelines for the prevention of intravascular catheter-related infections. The Hospital Infection Control Practices Advisory Committee, Center for Disease Control and Prevention. Pediatrics 2002;110:e51.
[42] Pollack MM, Yeh TS, Ruttiman UE, Holbrook PR, Fields AI. Evaluation of pediatric intensive care. Crit Care Med 1984;12:376–83.
[43] Richards MJ, Edwards JR, Culver DH, Gaynes RP. Nosocomial infections in combined medical-surgical intensive care units in the United States. Infect Control Hosp Epidemiol 2000;21:510–5.
[44] Langley JM, Hanakowski M, Leblanc JC. Unique epidemiology of nosocomial urinary tract infection in children. Am J Infect Control 2001;29:94–8.
[45] Pearson ML. Guideline for prevention of intravascular device-related infections: Part I. intravascular device-related infections: an overview. The Hospital Infection Control Practices Advisory Committee. Am J Infect Control 1996;24:262–77.
[46] Darouiche RO, Raad II, Heard SO, et al. A comparison of two antimicrobial-impregnated central venous catheters. Catheter Study Group. N Engl J Med 1999;340:1–8.
[47] McConnell SA, Gubbins PO, Anaissie EJ. Are antimicrobial-impregnated catheters effective? Replace the water and grab your washcloth, because we have a baby to wash. Clin Infect Dis 2004;39:1829–33.
[48] Elward AM, Warren DK, Fraser VJ. Ventilator-associated pneumonia in pediatric intensive care unit patients: risk factors and outcomes. Pediatrics 2002;109:758–64.
[49] Yogaraj JS, Elward AM, Fraser VJ. Rate, risk factors, and outcomes of nosocomial primary bloodstream infection in pediatric intensive care unit patients. Pediatrics 2002;110:481–5.
[50] Nataro JP, Corcoran L, Zirin S, et al. Prospective analysis of coagulase-negative staphylococcal infection in hospitalized infants. J Pediatr 1994;125:798–804.
[51] Tablan OC, Anderson LJ, Besser R, Bridges C, Hajjeh R. Guidelines for preventing health-care–associated pneumonia, 2003: recommendations of CDC and the Healthcare Infection Control Practices Advisory Committee. MMWR Recomm Rep 2004;53:1–36.

[52] Berman SA, Balkany TJ, Simmons MA. Otitis media in the neonatal intensive care unit. Pediatrics 1978;62:198–201.
[53] Guerin JM, Lustman C, Meyer P, Barbotin-Larrieau F. Nosocomial sinusitis in pediatric intensive care patients. Crit Care Med 1990;18:902.
[54] Gauvin F, Dassa C, Chaibou M, Proulx F, Farrell CA, Lacroix J. Ventilator-associated pneumonia in intubated children: comparison of different diagnostic methods. Pediatr Crit Care Med 2003;4:437–43.
[55] Pugin J, Auckenthaler R, Mili N, Janssens JP, Lew PD, Suter PM. Diagnosis of ventilator-associated pneumonia by bacteriologic analysis of bronchoscopic and nonbronchoscopic "blind" bronchoalveolar lavage fluid. Am Rev Respir Dis 1991;143:1121–9.
[56] Chastre J, Wolff M, Fagon JY, et al. Comparison of 8 vs 15 days of antibiotic therapy for ventilator-associated pneumonia in adults: a randomized trial. JAMA 2003;290:2588–98.
[57] Apisarnthanarak A, Holzmann-Pazgal G, Hamvas A, Olsen MA, Fraser VJ. Ventilator-associated pneumonia in extremely preterm neonates in a neonatal intensive care unit: characteristics, risk factors, and outcomes. Pediatrics 2003;112:1283–9.
[58] Davies HD, Jones EL, Sheng RY, Leslie B, Matlow AG, Gold R. Nosocomial urinary tract infections at a pediatric hospital. Pediatr Infect Dis J 1992;11:349–54.
[59] Lohr JA, Donowitz LG, Sadler JE 3rd. Hospital-acquired urinary tract infection. Pediatrics 1989;83:193–9.
[60] Wong ES. Guideline for prevention of catheter-associated urinary tract infections. Am J Infect Control 1983;11:28–36.
[61] Brook I. Microbiology and management of post-surgical wounds infection in children. Pediatr Rehabil 2002;5:171–6.
[62] Porras-Hernandez JD, Vilar-Compte D, Cashat-Cruz M, Ordorica-Flores RM, Bracho-Blanchet E, Avila-Figueroa C. A prospective study of surgical site infections in a pediatric hospital in Mexico City. Am J Infect Control 2003;31:302–8.
[63] Odio C, McCracken GH Jr, Nelson JD. CSF shunt infections in pediatrics: a seven-year experience. Am J Dis Child 1984;138:1103–8.
[64] Diagnostic standards and classification of tuberculosis in adults and children. This official statement of the American Thoracic Society and the Centers for Disease Control and Prevention was adopted by the ATS Board of Directors, July 1999. This statement was endorsed by the Council of the Infectious Disease Society of America, September 1999. Am J Respir Crit Care Med 2000;161:1376–95.
[65] Siegel JD. Controversies in isolation and general infection control practices in pediatrics. Semin Pediatr Infect Dis 2002;13:48–54.
[66] Gelber SE, Ratner AJ. Hospital-acquired viral pathogens in the neonatal intensive care unit. Semin Perinatol 2002;26:346–56.
[67] Soule H, Genoulaz O, Gratacap-Cavallier B, et al. Monitoring rotavirus environmental contamination in a pediatric unit using polymerase chain reaction. Infect Control Hosp Epidemiol 1999;20:432–4.
[68] Widdowson MA, van Doornum GJ, van der Poel WH, et al. An outbreak of diarrhea in a neonatal medium care unit caused by a novel strain of rotavirus: investigation using both epidemiologic and microbiological methods. Infect Control Hosp Epidemiol 2002;23: 665–70.
[69] Nakata S, Adachi N, Ukae S, et al. Outbreaks of nosocomial rotavirus gastro-enteritis in a paediatric ward. Eur J Pediatr 1996;155:954–8.
[70] Barnes GL, Callaghan SL, Kirkwood CD, Bogdanovic-Sakran N, Johnston LJ, Bishop RF. Excretion of serotype G1 rotavirus strains by asymptomatic staff: a possible source of nosocomial infection. J Pediatr 2003;142:722–5.
[71] Thorburn K, Kerr S, Taylor N, van Saene HK. RSV outbreak in a paediatric intensive care unit. J Hosp Infect 2004;57:194–201.

[72] Steele AD, Mnisi YN, Williams MM, Bos P, Aspinall S. Electrophoretic typing of nosocomial rotavirus infection in a general paediatric unit showing the continual introduction of community strains. J Med Virol 1993;40:126–32.
[73] Macartney KK, Gorelick MH, Manning ML, Hodinka RL, Bell LM. Nosocomial respiratory syncytial virus infections: the cost-effectiveness and cost-benefit of infection control. Pediatrics 2000;106:520–6.
[74] Archibald L, Phillips L, Monnet D, McGowan JE Jr, Tenover F, Gaynes R. Antimicrobial resistance in isolates from inpatients and outpatients in the United States: increasing importance of the intensive care unit. Clin Infect Dis 1997;24:211–5.
[75] Ghaffar F, Friedland IR, Katz K, et al. Increased carriage of resistant non-pneumococcal alpha-hemolytic streptococci after antibiotic therapy. J Pediatr 1999;135:618–23.
[76] Sattler CA, Mason EO Jr, Kaplan SL. Prospective comparison of risk factors and demographic and clinical characteristics of community-acquired, methicillin-resistant versus methicillin-susceptible *Staphylococcus aureus* infection in children. Pediatr Infect Dis J 2002; 21:910–7.
[77] Grohskopf LA, Sinkowitz-Cochran RL, Garrett DO, et al. A national point-prevalence survey of pediatric intensive care unit-acquired infections in the United States. J Pediatr 2002;140:432–8.
[78] Shah SS, Sinkowitz-Cochran RL, Keyserling HL, Jarvis WR. Vancomycin use in pediatric cardiothoracic surgery patients. Pediatr Infect Dis J 1999;18:558–60.
[79] Shah SS, Sinkowitz-Cochran RL, Keyserling HL, Jarvis WR. Vancomycin use in pediatric neurosurgery patients. Am J Infect Control 1999;27:482–7.
[80] Sinkowitz RL, Keyserling H, Walker TJ, Holland J, Jarvis WR. Epidemiology of vancomycin usage at a children's hospital, 1993 through 1995. Pediatr Infect Dis J 1997; 16:485–9.
[81] de Man P, Verhoeven BA, Verbrugh HA, Vos MC, van den Anker JN. An antibiotic policy to prevent emergence of resistant bacilli. Lancet 2000;355:973–8.
[82] Toltzis P, Yamashita T, Vilt L, et al. Antibiotic restriction does not alter endemic colonization with resistant gram-negative rods in a pediatric intensive care unit. Crit Care Med 1998;26:1893–9.
[83] Toltzis P, Dul MJ, Hoyen C, et al. The effect of antibiotic rotation on colonization with antibiotic-resistant bacilli in a neonatal intensive care unit. Pediatrics 2002;110:707–11.
[84] Gross R, Morgan AS, Kinky DE, Weiner M, Gibson GA, Fishman NO. Impact of a hospital-based antimicrobial management program on clinical and economic outcomes. Clin Infect Dis 2001;33:289–95.
[85] Muto CA, Jernigan JA, Ostrowsky BE, et al. SHEA guideline for preventing nosocomial transmission of multidrug-resistant strains of *Staphylococcus aureus* and enterococcus. Infect Control Hosp Epidemiol 2003;24:362–86.
[86] Georgantopulos R, Dubberke E, Reno H, et al. Risk factors for *Staphylococcus aureus* nasal colonization among patients newly admitted to multiple hospitals. Presented at Society for Healthcare Epidemiology of America, Los Angeles, 2005.

ELSEVIER
SAUNDERS

Infect Dis Clin N Am 19 (2005) 667–689

INFECTIOUS
DISEASE CLINICS
OF NORTH AMERICA

The Link Between Bronchiolitis and Asthma

Tuomas Jartti, MD[a], Mika J. Mäkelä, MD[b], Timo Vanto, MD[a], Olli Ruuskanen, MD[a,*]

[a]*Department of Pediatrics, Turku University Hospital, PO Box 52, FIN-20520 Turku, Finland*
[b]*Department of Pediatrics, Skin and Allergy Hospital, Helsinki University Hospital, PO Box 160, FIN-00029 HUS, Finland*

Bronchiolitis is a lower respiratory tract infection of young children. Clinical features include expiratory wheezing, tachypnea, and hypoxia caused by obstruction of the small airways [1]. It has been suggested that the diagnosis of bronchiolitis would apply only to infants, but the use of the diagnosis varies greatly. In many clinical studies, all wheezing illnesses other than asthma in children younger than 3 years of age have been diagnosed as bronchiolitis. Asthma is a chronic inflammation of the airways, and clinically an acute asthma attack mimics bronchiolitis. The diagnosis of asthma should be used only after recurrent reversible wheezing episodes [2].

In the United States alone, an estimated 3% of all children are hospitalized for bronchiolitis in their first year of life, which is equivalent to more than 100,000 hospitalizations annually. Retrospective, hospital record–based studies have found that the prevalence of bronchiolitis increased in the 1980s and 1990s [3,4]. The prevalence of asthma also has increased—from 3.6% to 6.2% from 1980 to 1996. From 1997 to 2000, the prevalence of asthma attacks has remained unchanged, however, suggesting that the burden from childhood asthma may have plateaued [5].

The relationship between bronchiolitis and the development of asthma and atopy (ie, immediate-type hypersensitivity) has been studied for many years. The development of atopy is particularly interesting because the persistent form of asthma is mainly atopic. It has been estimated that 50% of children with bronchiolitis have recurrent wheezing (assessed by the parents) or asthma (diagnosed by a physician) during the following 2

The study was supported by the Turku University Foundation.
* Corresponding author.
E-mail address: olli.ruuskanen@tyks.fi (O. Ruuskanen).

0891-5520/05/$ - see front matter
doi:10.1016/j.idc.2005.05.010 *id.theclinics.com*

decades of life. The association between bronchiolitis and atopy defined as specific IgE antibodies or a positive skin prick test has been weak [6,7].

Genetics and environmental influences, such as respiratory viral infections and allergen exposure, are associated closely with airway hyperreactivity. Respiratory viral infections predisposing to chronic asthma occur during infancy when immunologic maturation has not yet developed fully. It is crucial to understand how these different factors may contribute to the onset of asthma (Fig. 1). It is well established that respiratory syncytial virus (RSV) bronchiolitis is associated strongly with recurrent wheezing and asthma, at least during the first decade of life [7,8]. Preliminary findings suggest that rhinovirus-induced bronchiolitis is an even stronger risk factor and may be the first sign of asthma [9].

Viral etiology of bronchiolitis and asthma

Many respiratory viruses can cause bronchiolitis (Table 1). Many studies from the 1970s and 1980s have shown that RSV is the dominant causative agent, and it is virtually the only agent inducing epidemics. RSV infection has been detected in 50% to 70% of patients with bronchiolitis [10,12,14]. RSV is a rare pathogen in older hospitalized children [10,14] because nearly

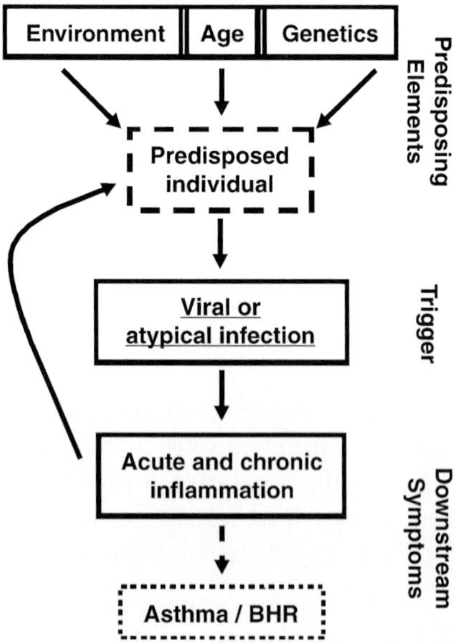

Fig. 1. Multifactorial influences on the development of asthma. BHR, bronchial hyperreactivity. (*From* Openshaw PJ, Yamaguchi Y, Tregoning JS. Childhood infections, the developing immune system, and the origins of asthma. J Allergy Clin Immunol 2004;114:1276; with permission.)

Table 1
Studies on viral etiology of bronchiolitis

Year of study[a]	Wheezing episodes/control subjects	Age (mo)	Viral identification rates (%)								
			RSV	Rhinovirus	Enteroviruses	Parainfluenza virus	Influenza virus	Adenovirus	Coronavirus	hMPV	Total positive
1999 [10]	22/17	<24	68/0	41/41[b]	1/0			0/1	0/1		82
2000 [11]	84	<12	54	19	12	0	0	13	0		74
2002 [12]	118	<18	53	21		3	3	8	3		74
2003 [9]	81	<24	26	33	12	14		5	0		73
2004 [13,14][c]	71	3–12	55	18	14	6	3	1	1	11	90
	179/17	3–36	36	21/0[d]	21/0[d]	5	2	5	2	7	87

Abbreviations: hMPV, human metapneumovirus; RSV, respiratory syncytial virus.

[a] Including studies using polymerase chain reaction with a sampling period of >1 year.

[b] With polymerase chain reaction; 23/25 using culture only.

[c] New subgroup analysis.

[d] Nontypable rhino-enterovirus: 15/18.

all children have been infected with RSV within the first 2 years of life, and a child's initial RSV infection is typically the most severe. RSV epidemics usually begin yearly in the late fall and peak in November to March. In some countries, such as Finland, RSV infections occur in double-humped outbreaks in 2-year cycles [1,14].

Studies using polymerase chain reaction (PCR) techniques have shown a prominent role for rhinovirus and enteroviruses in the etiology of acute bronchiolitis. Rhinovirus has been detected in 20% to 40% and enteroviruses in 10% to 20% of cases [10,14]. Rhinovirus bronchiolitis often occurs during RSV epidemics. The clinical value of positive picornavirus PCR test has been questioned because RNA of these viruses has been detected in 20% to 40% of asymptomatic children [10,13]. The authors have found that the degree of picornavirus PCR positivity markedly decreases over 2 to 3 weeks and disappears over 5 to 6 weeks after an acute wheezing episode, suggesting that positive picornavirus PCR is related to an acute symptomatic infection [13]. Rhinovirus outbreaks occur during the fall and spring, and enterovirus outbreaks usually occur only during the fall [14].

Viral respiratory infections commonly are associated with acute asthma (Table 2). Rhinovirus is the main trigger of exacerbations, associated with 30% to 80% of cases. The community study of Johnston et al [15] reported picornaviruses by PCR in half of the cases with decreased peak expiratory flow. Of these, 57% were confirmed as rhinovirus by culture. Two studies have focused on viral etiologies in young children with acute asthma [14,16]. Rhinovirus was found as an important viral agent in this patient group with a recovery rate of 27% to 44%.

In the authors' study, enteroviruses, which according to their name replicate most prolifically in the gastrointestinal tract, were related to acute asthma in 38% of the cases [14]. This finding is in agreement with the report of Rawlinson et al [17], who found enteroviruses by PCR in 29% of young children with well-documented asthma occurring in summer. Coronavirus has been found in 2% to 13% of children with acute exacerbations of asthma [10,14–16]. Other viruses account for 10% or less of the cases. Influenza viruses, which yearly circulate in the community, are less important. RSV is a rare causative agent of acute asthma in children older than age 2 years.

Pathogenesis of bronchiolitis

The major risk factors for bronchiolitis include young age, passive smoke exposure, small lung size, a chronic underlying condition, and having older siblings [18,19]. Genetic background also may influence the response to RSV infection because factors such as the polymorphisms of interleukin (IL)-8, IL-4, and its receptor and the surfactant protein D have been implicated in disease susceptibility and severity [20–23].

Table 2
Studies on viral etiology of acute asthma

Year of study[a]	Wheezing episodes/ control subjects	Age (y)	Viral identification rates (%) RSV	Rhinovirus	Enteroviruses	Parainfluenza virus	Influenza A/B virus	Adenovirus	Coronavirus	hMPV	Total positive
1995 [15]	161	9–11	4	50[b]		7	7		13		80[c]
1999 [10][d]	48/42	2–16	6/0	71/36[e]	2/0		2/0	2/0	6/0		83
1999 [16]	71	≤2	24	44	10[f]	4[f]	10[f]	5[f]	5[f]		86
	61	>2	18	51							77
2003 [17]	179	0.1–17	7	79		1	2			2	88
2004 [13,14][g]	49/17	0.4–3	22	27/0	33/0	4	4	12	0	0	90
	65/25	3–16	8	31/0[h]	38/0[h]	9	2	2	2	0	91

Abbreviations: hMPV, human metapneumovirus; RSV, respiratory syncytial virus.

[a] Including studies using polymerase chain reaction with a sampling period of >1 year.

[b] Number is for picornaviruses, of which 57% were rhinoviruses, the remaining viruses could not be cultured and were classified as rhinoviruses because most enteroviruses culture easily.

[c] In reported falls in peak expiratory flow.

[d] Children with wheezing were included. Excluded were children with bronchopulmonary dysplasia or using corticosteroids within the previous week.

[e] With polymerase chain reaction; 18/24% using culture only.

[f] Information not available of different age groups.

[g] New subgroup analyses.

[h] Nontypable rhino-enterovirus: 12/18 in children age <3 y and 17/12 in children age ≥3 y.

The viral infection begins with viruses infecting airway epithelial cells, which are the primary site of replication. Numerous cytokines and chemokines are produced, which recruit and activate inflammatory cells. Innate and adaptive immune responses are triggered. The damaged airway together with an antiviral response causes epithelial edema and increased mucus production and vascular permeability. These events lead to narrowing of small bronchioles and consequent airway dysfunction and wheezing.

RSV infection activates signaling pathways in airway epithelium through a toll-like receptor 4 and by the generation of oxidative stress [24,25]. Host cell recognition of viral RNA produced by viral replication initiates antiviral and proinflammatory responses within the cell. When newly synthesized viruses are released into the airway, the antiviral response is enhanced by mononuclear cells. Monocytes, macrophages, and probably dendritic cells secrete proinflammatory cytokines, such as IL-1, IL-8, tumor necrosis factor (TNF)-α, and interferon (IFN)-α, which further activate other cells and induce adhesion molecules. Because most recruited cells are neutrophils, it has been suggested that neutrophils and their activation products are important in the causation of airway obstruction. A few recruited cells are mononuclear cells and eosinophils. Lymphocytes also are recruited into the airways during the early stages of infection and are probably important in limiting the extent of infection and clearing virus-infected cells. Th1 and Th2 type responses have been implicated in infants with RSV bronchiolitis [26].

Most rhinoviruses are recognized by the intercellular adhesion molecule 1 (ICAM-1) [27,28]. The rhinovirus-induced antiviral response, as in the case in RSV infection, is considered to be responsible for the clinical symptoms. The antiviral response to rhinovirus infection includes type 1 interferons and nitric oxide and the production of cytokines and chemokines, such as IL-1α/β, IL-8, IL-10, TNF-α, granulocyte-macrophage colony-stimulating factor, epithelial neutrophil-activating protein-78, RANTES (regulated on activation, normal T cell expressed and secreted), eotaxin 1/2, macrophage-inflammatory proteins, and leukotrienes, which influence the subsequent innate and specific immune response. Interferons are especially important in antiviral response because they are potent activators of antiviral effector cells as natural killer cells, CD8 T lymphocytes, and macrophages. The cellular response is mainly neutrophilic, but mast cells and eosinophils also infiltrate the infection site. Bronchial mucosal eosinophilic infiltrates have been found in biopsy specimens from healthy and asthmatic volunteers during an experimental rhinovirus infection [29]. The accumulation of eosinophils is influenced by IL-5, granulocyte-macrophage colony-stimulating factor, IL-8, RANTES, and eotaxin [27]. All of these except IL-5 have been produced by airway epithelial cells in vitro after a rhinovirus infection.

So far, only one report has been published comparing virus-specific inflammatory cell responses in bronchiolitis patients age younger than 2 years. According to Korppi et al [30], children with rhinovirus infection compared with children with RSV infection were older and presented more often with atopic dermatitis and blood eosinophilia. The groups did not differ in total serum IgE. Similarly, the authors have found a mean peripheral blood eosinophil count of 0.11×10^9/L and a neutrophil count of 3.48×10^9/L in children age younger than 2 years with the first wheezing attack induced by RSV, whereas in children with picornavirus bronchiolitis, the corresponding counts were 0.42×10^9/L and 5.87×10^9/L (unpublished findings). Although it is impossible to determine whether these differences are due to the virus, or whether they are related to a preexisting inflammation, there are great cellular differences in the courses of rhinovirus and RSV bronchiolitis. Eosinophilia and even neutrophilia in the peripheral blood are associated more clearly with rhinovirus bronchiolitis than RSV bronchiolitis.

Genetics of airway hyperreactivity

A parental history of childhood respiratory problems is an important risk factor for infantile lower respiratory tract illnesses. In the Tucson Children's Respiratory Study, the greatest risk was early onset of the parental illness [31]. A parental history of asthma or bronchiolitis with onset before age 3 years was associated with wheezing illnesses in offspring. The continuation of wheezing from early life until age 6 years also has a clear association with a maternal history of asthma and atopy [18]. Although these findings suggest a familial component in childhood wheezing, epidemiologic studies do not answer the question whether the risk is inherited genetically.

Since the 1990s, significant progress has been made in identifying the genes responsible for the development of asthma and atopy [32–34]. There are probably many susceptibility genes that act either alone or in combination with other genes increasing the risk of the disease [35]. Genetic studies are confounded by influences of genetic heterogeneity, heterogeneous phenotypes of asthma among the studied subjects, incomplete or low penetrance (despite a relatively high prevalence), and genotype-environment and gene-gene interactions [32,36].

Reviews of genetic association studies have linked 60 genes to asthma [33,34]. Of these, more than 30 have been replicated at least once, but less than 10 have been replicated in five or more studies. Many previous studies of the genetics of asthma have been criticized for being underpowered in view of the relatively modest effects of the individual genes. Nonreplicated studies may represent false-positive findings. Four interesting candidate genes have been highlighted in asthma, however. A role has been suggested for *ADAM33* in airway remodeling and smooth muscle reactivity; for *PHF11,* in immunoregulation, especially that of B lymphocytes; for *DPP10,* in cytokine processing, especially in T cells; and for *GPRA,* in bronchial epithelial and smooth muscle surface receptor functions. Although it is difficult to separate atopy and bronchial hyperreactivity because of similarities in their regulatory networks, a definite genetic effect occurs in the two diseases.

Genetic predisposition to strong proinflammatory or weak anti-inflammatory capacity may increase the risk for atopic diseases. Regulatory T cells, which mediate their effects through anti-inflammatory cytokines, such as IL-10 and transforming growth factor-β, are able to suppress Th1 and Th2 cells [37]. Lower levels of IL-10 and transforming growth factor-β have been reported in asthmatic and atopic individuals [38,39], whereas proinflammatory cytokines, such as the IL-1α genotype, have been more frequent in atopic subjects [40]. The matter is still controversial, however [41]. IL-10 responses have been highly influenced by viral infections in atopic asthmatics, and the responses in infants also seem to be different from responses in adults [42,43].

Environmental influences on the immunopathogenesis of atopic asthma

Atopy and asthma may not be explained simply by the Th1/Th2 paradigm or abnormal proinflammatory or anti-inflammatory capacity, as suggested in a report by Heaton et al [36]. These investigators showed mixed Th1/Th2 immune responses in wheezing children. Although they confirmed that allergic diseases and asthma are associated with Th2 production (IL-5, eosinophilia, IgE production), they also showed that IFN-γ was associated with increased immediate skin test reactivity and with airway hyperreactivity [36]. These findings are in agreement with findings from a mouse model, suggesting that Th1 responses could increase the severity of allergic diseases and asthma [44]. IL-10 has been found to have a protective effect inhibiting immediate skin test reactions, as also stated earlier, but it also is associated with airway hyperreactivity in children without allergies and may increase the severity of airway disease in these subjects. The diversity of these responses may indicate that atopy is influenced not only by genetic heterogeneity, but also environmental effects, such as infections or exposure to allergens, which occur with varying intensities in different individuals [45].

Since 1989, the scope of the hygiene hypothesis has extended to environmental microbial burdens in general and the regulation of the pattern of immune responses in early life [46,47]. Exposure to various environmental factors may influence inherited susceptibility to asthma and allergies by either increasing or decreasing the penetrance of predisposing genes. Interaction of viral infections in early life may be particularly important because RSV has been found to be an independent risk factor for the development of asthma [7,8,48], and a preliminary report suggests that this risk may be reduced by postponing the first RSV infection with RSV immunoglobulin [49]. IL-4 producing T cells responding to RSV and cat antigens have been reported to be more frequent in 7- and 8-year-old children with a history of RSV bronchiolitis [50], suggesting that early viral infection may affect Th2 polarization.

Repeated exposure to allergens may lead to the development of manifest atopy in early life, especially in immunologically susceptible individuals.

Exposure to allergen during the first 2 years of life has predicted asthma better than exposure later in childhood [51]. A prophylactic reduction of exposure to house dust mite from birth has reduced the risk for wheeze and subsequent sensitization at school age [52]. It has been suggested that no other major factors independent of atopic status determine persistent childhood asthma, defined as bronchial hyperreactivity [18,53]. In these children, symptoms can be produced with inhalation of allergen and reduced by moving the child to an allergen-free environment [54]. Respiratory viral infections are frequent triggers of acute bronchospasm also in allergic individuals, however [55]. Respiratory viral infections have been found to be more important seasonal triggers of exacerbations of asthma than pollen or spore counts [56].

Immunologic immaturity of infants

Human neonates exhibit decreased or aberrant innate, cellular, and humoral immune responses compared with adults. Many of the cells of the immune system are not intrinsically immature, but they lack the proper environmental influences to mount adult-type responses. The size of lymphocyte subpopulations shows marked changes during early life. The absolute number of B lymphocytes increases immediately after birth and remains unchanged until 2 years of age, then gradually decreases toward adult age. T lymphocytes increase after birth and decrease from 2 years to adulthood. Thymic involution starts at the age of 1 year and continues with a yearly loss of 3% [57]. The number of natural killer cells decreases over the first 2 months of life, then remains unchanged [58]. Cord blood has a decreased frequency of antigen-presenting dendritic cells, which present immunophenotypically with a higher degree of immaturity than adult dendritic cells [59]. Cord blood dendritic cells have a reduced ability to attain the mature adult phenotype and a reduced ability to activate naive $CD4^+$ T cells to produce IFN-γ, suggesting that they are intrinsically preprogrammed against the generation of Th1 immune response [60].

Functionally, neonatal T cells proliferate poorly in response to antigenic and allogeneic stimulation. Human neonatal T cells produce lower levels of Th1 and Th2 cytokines than adult cells. It is well established that cord blood cells respond more with Th2 cytokines (IL-4, IL-5, IL-9, IL-13) and less with Th1 cytokines (IFN-γ, IL-2, IL-12, TNF-α). Poor production of IFN-γ may be attributed to decreased production of IL-12 [61]. Neonatal CD8 T cells produce high levels of IL-13, which may account for the type 2 bias [62]. It was reported that compared with adults, neonates have immature IL-10 and IFN-γ responses [63]. The neonatal Th1 response may not always be poorer than the adult Th1 response, but also can be dependent on the antigen [64].

During the first year of life, maternal IgG is replaced by neonatal IgM, IgG, and IgA. Many studies have shown that the primary T cell–dependent antibody response in the neonatal period is weak. Clinically, it is seen as a poor response to polysaccharide antigens. In a large study of 23-valent pneumococcal polysaccharide vaccine, poor antibody responses and no clinical protection were detected in children younger than 6 months of age [65]. A poor response to polysaccharide antigens coincides with the lack of marginal–zone $CD21^{+}$ B cells and a high rate of cells coexpressing IgM and IgD [66].

Postnatal development of human immune responses is inadequately studied, but several single observations support the view that the human immune response mainly matures to the adult level during the first 2 years of life. B lymphocytes produce immunoglobulin levels close to adult levels, and the levels of lymphocyte subpopulations stabilize. The response to polysaccharide antigens can be detected in children older than age 2 years, and at the same age the histologic structure of the spleen is adult-type [66,67]. By 1 year of age, almost all Vδ1 T cells in blood have activated and changed to memory T cells, reflecting immunologic maturation [68]. Mucosal immunity, immature at birth, usually develops fully in the first year of life [69]. It was reported that the recruitment of inflammatory cells to the nose is at full potential at age 2 years. The number of nasal Th2 driving (IL-4) and regulatory (IL-10) cytokine-positive cells has been found to decrease over the first 24 months of life [70].

All these observations support the view that the immune system is immature for the first 1 to 2 years of life and may be susceptible to delayed or permanent change induced by environmental factors, such as viral infections. It has been suggested that delayed maturation of immune responses may be a risk factor for allergies and asthma [71].

A neonatal mouse model has supported this hypothesis, showing that age at the first RSV infection determines the pattern of disease during reinfection in adulthood. The strongest Th2 responses were seen in mice primed at 1 day of age. Neonatal priming was followed by severe disease and an increased inflammatory cell response during reinfection at 12 weeks. Delayed priming led to less severe disease and enhanced IFN-γ production. RSV infection at a very young age has the potential to cause long-term alterations in the immune system [72]. It has been suggested further that chronicity or persistence of pathogens in the lung may perpetuate the inflammation, which is exacerbated by new infections [73]. This persistent inflammation drives the airway reactivity characteristic of asthma.

Development of recurrent wheezing and asthma after bronchiolitis

Long-term prospective studies have shown a link between bronchiolitis and asthma (Table 3). In a study from the United Kingdom, Noble et al [82] monitored a cohort of 101 hospitalized infants with acute bronchiolitis (66% RSV positive) and 47 control infants. Abnormal pulmonary function still was found 9 to 10 years after hospitalization. Forced expiratory flow in 1 second (FEV_1) and peak expiratory flow were 5% to 9% lower than in controls. Two to three times more episodes of wheeze and diagnosed asthma were reported in index children than in controls. The history of bronchiolitis was the only variable related to wheezing and diagnosis of asthma. Virus-specific (RSV positive or negative) analysis was not reported. No differences were found in histamine challenge and skin prick tests.

The Tucson Children's Respiratory Study followed a large cohort of children from birth to 13 years of age [7]. Although bronchiolitis was not confirmed by a physician in all cases, RSV lower respiratory tract illnesses were associated with an increased risk of frequent wheeze by age 6. The risk decreased markedly with age and was not significant by age 13. The index cases had a lower FEV_1 than controls, but no difference was seen in the bronchodilator response. RSV lower respiratory tract illness was not related to atopic status on the basis of skin prick tests or serum IgE concentrations.

In a Swedish study, 47 hospitalized RSV-positive infants were followed for 13 years, and the last interim analyses were performed at age 7 years [8,48]. The cumulative prevalence of asthma was 10 times higher, and the cumulative prevalence of any wheezing was almost twice more common in index cases than in controls at age 7 years. Allergic sensitization also was found almost twice more common in RSV children than in control subjects. At age 13 years, the occurrence of symptoms over the previous 12 months for asthma or recurrent wheezing was still more than five times higher in the RSV group than among the controls. RSV bronchiolitis had the highest independent risk ratio for current asthma. At this age, only borderline significance was found for sensitization to common inhaled allergens, however. Any positivity in skin prick tests or specific serum IgE concentrations did not show any difference, whereas dander-specific or pollen-specific tests showed a significant difference.

The longest prospective follow-up period of 19 years was reported in a Finnish study, which included 54 children hospitalized for bronchiolitis and 45 controls [85]. Two definitions for asthma were used: physician-diagnosed asthma and previously diagnosed asthma with recent asthmatic symptoms (physician-diagnosed asthma included). By these two definitions, asthma was present in 30% and 41% in the bronchiolitis group and in 11% in the control group. Lower baseline pulmonary function (ie, FEV_1, FEV_1/forced vital capacity, midexpiratory flow at 25% and 50% of forced vital capacity) was found in index cases, but no difference was seen on methacholine inhalation challenge. No significant difference was found in the prevalence of positive skin prick test reactions to common inhalant allergens. Sensitization to cat and dog dander was more than twice more common, however, in the bronchiolitis group than in the control group. The earlier studies reported a link between bronchiolitis and physician-defined asthma and abnormal pulmonary function occurring for 19 years [85]. For RSV bronchiolitis only, the link has been found to last for 13 years for

Table 3
Important long-term studies of the link between bronchiolitis and reactive airway disease

First author[a]	Year	Design	No. patients/controls	Age on entry (mo)	Viral etiology (%)		Follow-up time (y)	End points and results: patients versus controls (odds ratio, 95% CI *P* value)			
					RSV	Other		Recurrent wheezing	Physician-diagnosed asthma	Abnormal pulmonary function test	Atopy[b]
Sims [74]	1978	Ret	35/35	<12	100[c]		8	51% vs 3% ($P < .001$)[d]		PEF 237 L/mm vs 265 L/min ($P < .02$)	NS
Pullan [75]	1982	Ret	130/111	<12 (mean 4)	100[c]		10	42% vs 19% ($P < .001$)[d]	NS	Exercise test or histamine challenge positive 25% vs 7% ($P < .001$)	NS
Mok [76]	1982	Ret	200/200	<12 (mean 4)	50[c]		7	47% vs 17% ($P < .01$)[d]; 11% vs 1% ($P < .01$)[e]	9% vs 2.5% ($P < .05$)[d]	FEV_1 91% vs 95% predicted ($P < .005$), >10% fall after exercise 53% vs 37% ($P < .05$)	
McConnochie [77]	1984	Ret	59/177	<24			8	44% vs 14% ($P < 0.001$)[e]	25% vs 7% ($P < 0.001$)[d], 19% vs 4% ($P < 0.001$)[e]		
McConnochie [78]	1985	Ret	25/25	<24			8–12			FEF_{25-75} baseline 64% vs 75% predicted ($P = .04$), after cold air −9.0% vs −15.7% ($P = .04$)	
McConnochie [79]	1989	Ret	51/102	<24			13	NS	NS		
Carlsen [80]	1987	Pro	51/24	<1	61	6[f]	2	No. episodes, median 3 vs 0 ($P < .01$)			NS

Osundwa [81]	1993	Ret	70/70	Mean 4 (range 3–8)	100[c]		2	44% vs 12.9% ($P = .001$)[d]			
Noble [82]	1997	Pro	61/47	Mean 4 (range 1–12)	66		9–10	34% vs 13% (3.6, 1.3–9.8, $P = .018$)[d]	39% vs 13% (4.4, 1.6–12, $P = .004$)[e]	Baseline PEF 93% vs 102% predicted (95% CI of differences 4.1–13.4, $P < .001$), FEV_1 91% vs 96% predicted (0.5–9.6, $P = .03$)	NS
Stein [7]	1999	Pro	68/669 56/545 79/634 49/469	<36	44	28[g]	6 8 11 13	Year 11: RSV 2.4, 1.3–4.6, $P \leq .01$[d]; Year 13: other virus 3.1, 1.3–7.6, $P \leq .01$[d]; negative test 2.1, 1–4.3, $P \leq .05$[d]		Year 11: RSV FEV_1 baseline 2.1, 2.1–2.2, $P \leq .001$; negative test 2.1, 2.1–2.2, $P \leq .05$	NS
Weber [83]	1999	Pro	105/105	Median 4 (quartiles 2–6)			3	10% vs 1%[e] (IRR 7.4, 5.1–17.5)[d]			
Kneyber [84]	2000	Meta-analysis[h]	117/163	<12	0–100		<5	<5 y: 36% vs 6% (5.5, 2.4–12.6)[d]; ≥5 y: 6% vs 3% (2.4, 0.7–8.4)[d]			NS
			230/321	<12			≥5				
Kotaniemi-Syrjänen [9]	2003	Pro	44	1–24	23[c]	45[c,i]	6		4.1, 1–16.8 ($P = .047$)[j]		NS

(*continued on next page*)

Table 3 (*continued*)

First author[a]	Year	Design	No. patients/controls	Age on entry (mo)	Viral etiology (%)		Follow-up time (y)	End points and results: patients versus controls (odds ratio, 95% CI P value)			
					RSV	Other		Recurrent wheezing	Physician-diagnosed asthma	Abnormal pulmonary function test	Atopy[b]
Sigurs [8,48]	2000 2004	Pro	47/93	<12 (mean 4)	100[c]		7 13	Year 7: 68% vs 34% ($P < .001$)[d] Year 13: NS	Year 13: 37% vs 5.4% ($P < .001$)[d], 28% vs 3.3% ($P < .001$)[e]	Year 13: baseline FEV_1/FVC 85% vs 88% predicted ($P = .001$), after β_2-agonist 88% vs 89% predicted ($P = .043$), fall in FEV_1 after dry air hyperventilation 6.1% vs 4.6% ($P = .047$), reversibility NS	Year 7: 41% vs 22% ($P = .039$) Year 13: NS[k]
Piippo-Savolainen [85]	2004	Pro	54/45	Median 10 (range 1–24)			19		30% vs 11% (3.4, 1.1–10.1)[e,l]	Abnormal pulmonary function 36% vs 11% (4.5, 1.5–13.2)[l]	NS[k]

Abbreviations: FEF_{25-75}, forced expiratory flow at 25–75% range; FEV_1, forced expiratory flow in 1 second; IRR, incidence rate ratio; NS, nonsignificant; PEF, peak expiratory flow; Pro, prospective; Ret, retrospective; RSV, respiratory syncytial virus.

[a] Only the last positive reports are included of studies with many interim analyses.

[b] Confirmed by specific IgE antibodies or skin prick test.

[c] Inclusion criteria.

[d] Cumulative.

[e] Currently or previous year.

[f] Parainfluenza $n = 2$ (4%), rhinovirus $n = 1$ (2%).

[g] Parainfluenza $n = 68$ (14%), other viruses $n = 68$ (14%) (including adenovirus, influenza virus, cytomegalovirus, rhinovirus, bacterial and mixed infections), negative test $n = 129$ (27%).

[h] Including [75,76,79,86].

[i] Rhinovirus $n = 20$ and virus negative $n = 14$.

[j] Between rhinovirus-positive and rhinovirus-negative cases.

[k] For any test positive.

[l] Comparison included pneumonia group, which is not shown.

physician-defined asthma [8]. No studies have reported a convincing link between bronchiolitis and current atopy after age 7 years.

Only two studies have evaluated the role of bronchiolitis induced by other viruses. Kotaniemi-Syrjanen et al [9] compared the development of asthma after RSV and rhinovirus bronchiolitis. An average of 6 years later, asthma was present in 10% of the RSV group subjects compared with 60% of the rhinovirus group subjects [9]. Although no significant difference was found, probably owing to small sample size, the difference was significant between rhinovirus-positive and rhinovirus-negative cases. The authors have confirmed the finding in a 1-year follow-up of hospitalized children after their first bout of bronchiolitis. Asthma (ie, three physician-verified wheezing attacks within 12 months) was diagnosed in 21% of children after an RSV infection and in 64% of children after rhinovirus infection [87]. These findings encourage a more critical approach to the earlier study of Stein et al [7]. They reported that RSV lower respiratory tract illness is an independent risk factor for the subsequent development of wheezing up to age 11 years, but not age 13. Stein et al [7] also reported, but did not adequately discuss, the finding that at age 13 years there still was a significant link between bronchiolitis and asthma in the groups of children with other virus or with negative microbiology. At age 11 years, the negative group also had lower FEV_1 values. Rhinoviruses were not searched for by PCR techniques, and most of them probably were missed.

In addition to limited viral diagnostics, none of the aforementioned studies used or reported eosinophilia, which predicts the development of asthma, as an inclusion criterion or end point [88,89]. Further limitations of earlier studies include the variable diagnostic criteria for bronchiolitis and asthma. Six studies have extended the age range of bronchiolitis over 12 months. The older the children are, the more likely they are to exhibit characteristics predisposing for persistent wheezing, such as eosinophilia, atopy, and rhinovirus infection [30]. The most common end points were recurrent wheezing reported by the parents and clinically diagnosed asthma, which are not reliable assessments and may overestimate lung impairment [2,90]. Objective measurement of pulmonary function and physician-confirmed recurrent episodes of wheeze with a bronchodilator response are necessary for the diagnosis of asthma. Although baseline pulmonary function on follow-up is slightly decreased in the bronchiolitis groups of many studies, only two studies have shown evidence for bronchial hyperreactivity, characteristic of asthma [75,78]. When considering the results of earlier studies and their limitations, a clear association can be seen between bronchiolitis and recurrent wheezing, but the association between bronchiolitis and atopic asthma is not yet convincing [91].

Rhinovirus-induced bronchiolitis may be a first sign of asthma, as suggested by Kotaniemi-Syrjanen et al [9]. In a cross-sectional emergency department study, rhinovirus-induced wheezing was associated most strongly with atopy and eosinophilia [10]. Children with rhinovirus bronchiolitis also have higher blood eosinophil counts than children with RSV, as discussed earlier [30,89]. Immunologic events related to Th2 polarization seem to be important predisposing factors not only to the development of asthma, but also to rhinovirus-induced bronchiolitis. The link between these diseases is more likely to be attributable to this suggested immunologic anomaly that precedes or is induced by rhinovirus bronchiolitis rather than to structural damage to the airway as a result of bronchiolitis [19]. The hypothesis that airway inflammation before virus inoculation may be a risk factor for an adverse response to rhinovirus is supported by findings from an experimental rhinovirus infection in young adults with mild asthma. The study of Zambrano et al [92] has shown that subjects with high levels of IgE had greater lower respiratory tract symptom scores during the initial 4 days of the infection than the low IgE group. These subjects also had higher total blood eosinophil counts at baseline, increased eosinophil cationic protein in their nasal washes, and higher levels of expired nitric oxide at baseline and during peak cold symptoms. In agreement, another study has shown that on histamine challenge after experimental rhinovirus infection, allergic adult subjects show higher airway reactivity than healthy controls [93].

Why is rhinovirus infection such a common trigger of asthma exacerbations? First, the answer may be related to the expression of ICAM-1 by epithelial cells. ICAM-1 mediates viral binding, host infection, and antiviral response, and it is up-regulated by airway inflammation, including the rhinovirus infection itself [94]. Because Th2 cells predominate within the asthmatic airways, Bianco et al [95] addressed the question by studying the effects of Th2-associated and Th1-associated cytokines and experimental rhinovirus infections on ICAM-1 expression in epithelial cells in vitro. Th2-associated cytokines (IL-4, IL-5, IL-10, and IL-13) increased the ICAM-1 expression of uninfected and rhinovirus-infected cells, and these effects were dominant over the effects of IFN-γ. Second, a rhinovirus infection generates various inflammatory mediators, which probably enhance the ongoing inflammatory response in asthmatic airways at least in some circumstances [96]. Many studies have shown that rhinovirus infection can enhance lower airway histamine responses and eosinophil recruitment after allergen exposure [24]. Third, and probably most important, a defective IFN-γ response may not be able to limit the extent of the infection to upper airways. Peripheral blood mononuclear cells from atopic asthmatics have produced lower levels of IFN-γ and higher levels of IL-4 and IL-10 in response to rhinovirus infection than the cells from healthy subjects [42]. An experimental rhinovirus infection in atopic subjects has shown an inverse relationship between precold rhinovirus-induced IFN-γ secretion from peripheral blood mononuclear cells and peak virus shedding after inoculation [97]. Similarly, stronger Th1 responses in sputum cells (higher IFN-γ-to-IL-5 mRNA ratio) during induced colds have been found to be associated with milder cold symptoms and more rapid clearance of the virus [98]. Finally, the generation of IFN-γ has correlated directly with lung function [99]. These results together could explain why individuals with airway inflammation characterized by Th2 polarization and consequently by eosinophilia show increased susceptibility to and morbidity from rhinovirus infections and the associated exacerbation of asthma symptoms. The elevated secretion of IL-10 owing to rhinovirus infection may reduce partially the effectiveness of inflammatory mechanisms necessary for viral clearance and exacerbate airway inflammation and increase hyperreactivity.

Do viral infections contribute to sensitization to allergens? This is another important question, which cannot be answered exhaustively. Animal studies using experimental influenza virus, parainfluenza virus, and RSV infections have provided evidence that respiratory viral infections increase allergic sensitization to inhaled allergens and subsequently enhance airway inflammation, responsiveness, and obstruction [100–103]. Respiratory viral infections have been shown to prevent tolerance induction and enhance IgE-mediated allergic sensitization to inhaled allergens when infection and sensitization have coincided. The possible mechanisms involve increased permeability of airway mucosa to allergens and the recruitment of dendritic cells to the respiratory epithelium. Consequently the sensitization could be facilitated by increased antigen uptake and more effective antigen presentation. It has been suggested that T cells, especially $CD8^+$ T cells, IL-4, IL-5, and eosinophils are important regulators triggering airway hyperresponsiveness. Similarly, certain human respiratory viral infections may increase the risk of allergic sensitization by providing a local IL-4-high environment, as RSV studies show [50]. Recurrent respiratory viral infections with allergen exposure may contribute significantly to the onset of atopic asthma, but the full extent of these effects in humans remains to be evaluated.

Summary

Respiratory viral infections are closely related to bronchiolitis and acute asthma. RSV is the major causative agent of bronchiolitis in young infants, whereas rhinovirus is an important trigger of asthma exacerbations, but also is recognized increasingly in slightly older children with bronchiolitis. Bronchiolitis is followed by recurrent wheezing or asthma in 5% to 50% of children during the first 2 decades of life. Preliminary data indicate that rhinovirus bronchiolitis is a more potent risk factor for school-age asthma than RSV bronchiolitis. The authors hypothesize that an important link between bronchiolitis and asthma is a person's susceptibility to certain lower respiratory tract viral infections, especially to rhinovirus infection. This susceptibility probably is related to the strong genetic component of atopy and possibly to eosinophilic airway inflammation response, which are likely not only to increase susceptibility, but also to exacerbate rhinovirus infection. The immature immune system of children age 1 to 2 years may increase susceptibility to respiratory viral infections, and their immature immune system may be vulnerable to permanent change induced by environmental factors, such as viral infections. Recurrent respiratory viral infections, especially with allergen exposure, may contribute markedly to airway inflammation, airway hyperreactivity, and inception of atopic asthma. Lower respiratory tract rhinovirus infection in early life may be a first sign of asthma by identifying individuals with an underlying immunologic anomaly that predisposes to the development of asthma. Further studies are, needed to confirm this hypothesis.

References

[1] Ruuskanen O, Ogra PL. Respiratory syncytial virus. Curr Probl Pediatr 1993;23:50–79.

[2] National Asthma Education and Prevention Program Expert Panel Report. Guidelines for the diagnosis and management of asthma: update on selected topics—2002. J Allergy Clin Immunol 2002;110:S141–219.

[3] Shay DK, Holman RC, Newman RD, Liu LL, Stout JW, Anderson LJ. Bronchiolitis-associated hospitalizations among US children, 1980–1996. JAMA 1999;282:1440–6.

[4] Langley JM, LeBlanc JC, Smith B, Wang EE. Increasing incidence of hospitalization for bronchiolitis among Canadian children, 1980–2000. J Infect Dis 2003;188:1764–7.

[5] Akinbami LJ, Schoendorf KC. Trends in childhood asthma: prevalence, health care utilization, and mortality. Pediatrics 2002;110:315–22.

[6] Forster J, Tacke U, Krebs H, et al. Respiratory syncytial virus infection: its role in aeroallergen sensitization during the first two years of life. Pediatr Allergy Immunol 1996;7: 55–60.

[7] Stein RT, Sherrill D, Morgan WJ, et al. Respiratory syncytial virus in early life and risk of wheeze and allergy by age 13 years. Lancet 1999;354:541–5.

[8] Sigurs N, Gustafsson PM, Bjarnason R, et al. Severe respiratory syncytial virus bronchiolitis in infancy and asthma and allergy at age 13. Am J Respir Crit Care Med 2005;171:137–41.

[9] Kotaniemi-Syrjänen A, Vainionpää R, Reijonen TM, Waris M, Korhonen K, Korppi M. Rhinovirus-induced wheezing in infancy—the first sign of childhood asthma? J Allergy Clin Immunol 2003;111:66–71.

[10] Rakes GP, Arruda E, Ingram JM, et al. Rhinovirus and respiratory syncytial virus in wheezing children requiring emergency care: IgE and eosinophil analyses. Am J Respir Crit Care Med 1999;159:785–90.

[11] Andreoletti L, Lesay M, Deschildre A, Lambert V, Dewilde A, Wattre P. Differential detection of rhinoviruses and enteroviruses RNA sequences associated with classical immunofluorescence assay detection of respiratory virus antigens in nasopharyngeal swabs from infants with bronchiolitis. J Med Virol 2000;61:341–6.

[12] Papadopoulos NG, Moustaki M, Tsolia M, et al. Association of rhinovirus infection with increased disease severity in acute bronchiolitis. Am J Respir Crit Care Med 2002;165: 1285–9.

[13] Jartti T, Lehtinen P, Vuorinen T, Koskenvuo M, Ruuskanen O. Persistence of rhinovirus and enterovirus RNA after acute respiratory illness in children. J Med Virol 2004;72:695–9.

[14] Jartti T, Lehtinen P, Vuorinen T, et al. Respiratory picornaviruses and respiratory syncytial virus as causative agents of acute expiratory wheezing in children. Emerg Infect Dis 2004; 10:1095–101.

[15] Johnston SL, Pattemore PK, Sanderson G, et al. Community study of role of viral infections in exacerbations of asthma in 9–11 year old children. BMJ 1995;310:1225–9.
[16] Freymuth F, Vabret A, Brouard J, et al. Detection of viral, *Chlamydia pneumoniae* and *Mycoplasma pneumoniae* infections in exacerbations of asthma in children. J Clin Virol 1999;13:131–9.
[17] Rawlinson WD, Waliuzzaman Z, Carter IW, Belessis YC, Gilbert KM, Morton JR. Asthma exacerbations in children associated with rhinovirus but not human metapneumovirus infection. J Infect Dis 2003;187:1314–8.
[18] Martinez FD, Wright AL, Taussig LM, Holberg CJ, Halonen M, Morgan WJ. Asthma and wheezing in the first six years of life. The Group Health Medical Associates. N Engl J Med 1995;332:133–8.
[19] Young S, O'Keeffe PT, Arnott J, Landau LI. Lung function, airway responsiveness, and respiratory symptoms before and after bronchiolitis. Arch Dis Child 1995;72:16–24.
[20] Hull J, Thomson A, Kwiatkowski D. Association of respiratory syncytial virus bronchiolitis with the interleukin 8 gene region in UK families. Thorax 2000;55:1023–7.
[21] Lahti M, Löfgren J, Marttila R, et al. Surfactant protein D gene polymorphism associated with severe respiratory syncytial virus infection. Pediatr Res 2002;51:696–9.
[22] Hoebee B, Rietveld E, Bont L, et al. Association of severe respiratory syncytial virus bronchiolitis with interleukin-4 and interleukin-4 receptor alpha polymorphisms. J Infect Dis 2003;187:2–11.
[23] Heinzmann A, Ahlert I, Kurz T, Berner R, Deichmann KA. Association study suggests opposite effects of polymorphisms within IL8 on bronchial asthma and respiratory syncytial virus bronchiolitis. J Allergy Clin Immunol 2004;114:671–6.
[24] Gern JE. Viral respiratory infection and the link to asthma. Pediatr Infect Dis J 2004;23: S78–86.
[25] Heidema J, Kimpen JLL, van Bleek GM. Pathogenesis of respiratory syncytial virus bronchiolitis: immunology and genetics. In: Kimpen JLL, Ramilo O, editors. Respiratory tract infections, pathogenesis and emerging strategies for control. Norfolk: Horizon Bioscience; 2004. p. 233–52.
[26] Tripp RA, Moore D, Barskey A 4th, et al. Peripheral blood mononuclear cells from infants hospitalized because of respiratory syncytial virus infection express T helper-1 and T helper-2 cytokines and CC chemokine messenger RNA. J Infect Dis 2002;185:1388–94.
[27] Message SD, Johnston SL. Host defense function of the airway epithelium in health and disease: clinical background. J Leukoc Biol 2004;75:5–17.
[28] Ruuskanen O, Hyypiä T. Rhinovirus: is it really a relevant pathogen? In: Kimpen JLL, Ramilo O, editors. Respiratory tract infections, pathogenesis and emerging strategies for control. Norfolk: Horizon Bioscience; 2004. p. 291–317.
[29] Fraenkel DJ, Bardin PG, Sanderson G, Lampe F, Johnston SL, Holgate ST. Lower airways inflammation during rhinovirus colds in normal and in asthmatic subjects. Am J Respir Crit Care Med 1995;151:879–86.
[30] Korppi M, Kotaniemi-Syrjänen A, Waris M, Vainionpää R, Reijonen TM. Rhinovirus-associated wheezing in infancy: comparison with respiratory syncytial virus bronchiolitis. Pediatr Infect Dis J 2004;23:995–9.
[31] Camilli AE, Holberg CJ, Wright AL, Taussig LM. Parental childhood respiratory illness and respiratory illness in their infants. Group Health Medical Associates. Pediatr Pulmonol 1993;16:275–80.
[32] Steinke JW, Borish L, Rosenwasser LJ. Genetics of hypersensitivity. J Allergy Clin Immunol 2003;111:S495–501.
[33] Weiss ST, Raby BA. Asthma genetics 2003. Hum Mol Genet 2004;13:R83–9.
[34] Kere J, Laitinen T. Positionally cloned susceptibility genes in allergy and asthma. Curr Opin Immunol 2004;16:689–94.
[35] Xu J, Meyers DA, Ober C, et al. Collaborative Study on the Genetics of Asthma. Genomewide screen and identification of gene-gene interactions for asthma-susceptibility

loci in three US populations: collaborative study on the genetics of asthma. Am J Hum Genet 2001;68:1437–46.
[36] Heaton T, Rowe J, Turner S, et al. An immunoepidemiological approach to asthma: identification of in-vitro T-cell response patterns associated with different wheezing phenotypes in children. Lancet 2005;365:142–9.
[37] Akdis CA, Blesken T, Akdis M, Wuthrich B, Blaser K. Role of interleukin 10 in specific immunotherapy. J Clin Invest 1998;102:98–106.
[38] Borish L, Aarons A, Rumbyrt J, Cvietusa P, Negri J, Wenzel S. Interleukin-10 regulation in normal subjects and patients with asthma. J Allergy Clin Immunol 1996;97:1288–96.
[39] Arkwright PD, Chase JM, Babbage S, Pravica V, David TJ, Hutchinson IV. Atopic dermatitis is associated with a low-producer transforming growth factor beta(1) cytokine genotype. J Allergy Clin Immunol 2001;108:281–4.
[40] Karjalainen J, Hulkkonen J, Pessi T, et al. The IL1A genotype associates with atopy in nonasthmatic adults. J Allergy Clin Immunol 2002;110:429–34.
[41] Colavita AM, Hastie AT, Musani AI, et al. Kinetics of IL-10 production after segmental antigen challenge of atopic asthmatic subjects. J Allergy Clin Immunol 2000;106:880–6.
[42] Papadopoulos NG, Stanciu LA, Papi A, Holgate ST, Johnston SL. A defective type 1 response to rhinovirus in atopic asthma. Thorax 2002;57:328–32.
[43] van Benten IJ, van Drunen CM, Koevoet JL, et al. Reduced nasal IL-10 and enhanced TNFalpha responses during rhinovirus and RSV induced upper respiratory tract infection in atopic and non-atopic infants. J Med Virol 2005;75:348–57.
[44] Hansen G, Berry G, DeKruyff RH, Umetsu DT. Allergen-specific Th1 cells fail to counterbalance Th2 cell-induced airway hyperreactivity but cause severe airway inflammation. J Clin Invest 1999;103:175–83.
[45] Umetsu DT. Revising the immunological theories of asthma and allergy. Lancet 2005;365: 98–100.
[46] Strachan DP. Hay fever, hygiene, and household size. BMJ 1989;299:1259–60.
[47] Rautava S, Ruuskanen O, Ouwehand A, Salminen S, Isolauri E. The hygiene hypothesis of atopic disease—an extended version. J Pediatr Gastroenterol Nutr 2004;38:378–88.
[48] Sigurs N, Bjarnason R, Sigurbergsson F, Kjellman B. Respiratory syncytial virus bronchiolitis in infancy is an important risk factor for asthma and allergy at age 7. Am J Respir Crit Care Med 2000;161:1501–7.
[49] Wenzel SE, Gibbs RL, Lehr MV, Simoes EA. Respiratory outcomes in high-risk children 7 to 10 years after prophylaxis with respiratory syncytial virus immune globulin. Am J Med 2002;112:627–33.
[50] Pala P, Bjarnason R, Sigurbergsson F, Metcalfe C, Sigurs N, Openshaw PJ. Enhanced IL-4 responses in children with a history of respiratory syncytial virus bronchiolitis in infancy. Eur Respir J 2002;20:376–82.
[51] Sporik R, Holgate ST, Platts-Mills TA, Cogswell JJ. Exposure to house-dust mite allergen (Der p I) and the development of asthma in childhood: a prospective study. N Engl J Med 1990;323:502–7.
[52] Arshad SH, Bateman B, Matthews SM. Primary prevention of asthma and atopy during childhood by allergen avoidance in infancy: a randomised controlled study. Thorax 2003; 58:489–93.
[53] Sporik R, Ingram JM, Price W, Sussman JH, Honsinger RW, Platts-Mills TA. Association of asthma with serum IgE and skin test reactivity to allergens among children living at high altitude: tickling the dragon's breath. Am J Respir Crit Care Med 1995;151:1388–92.
[54] Platts-Mills TA, Rakes G, Heymann PW. The relevance of allergen exposure to the development of asthma in childhood. J Allergy Clin Immunol 2000;105:S503–8.
[55] Green RM, Custovic A, Sanderson G, Hunter J, Johnston SL, Woodcock A. Synergism between allergens and viruses and risk of hospital admission with asthma: case-control study. BMJ 2002;324:763.

[56] Carlsen KH, Orstavik I, Leegaard J, Hoeg H. Respiratory virus infections and aeroallergens in acute bronchial asthma. Arch Dis Child 1984;59:310–5.
[57] Steinmann GG. Changes in the human thymus during aging. Curr Top Pathol 1986;75: 43–88.
[58] Comans-Bitter WM, de Groot R, van den Beemd R, et al. Immunophenotyping of blood lymphocytes in childhood. Reference values for lymphocyte subpopulations. J Pediatr 1997;130:388–93.
[59] Crespo I, Paiva A, Couceiro A, Pimentel P, Orfao A, Regateiro F. Immunophenotypic and functional characterization of cord blood dendritic cells. Stem Cells Dev 2004;13:63–70.
[60] Langrish CL, Buddle JC, Thrasher AJ, Goldblatt D. Neonatal dendritic cells are intrinsically biased against Th-1 immune responses. Clin Exp Immunol 2002;128: 118–23.
[61] Marodi L. Down-regulation of Th1 responses in human neonates. Clin Exp Immunol 2002; 128:1–2.
[62] Ribeiro-do-Couto LM, Boeije LC, Kroon JS, et al. High IL-13 production by human neonatal T cells: neonate immune system regulator? Eur J Immunol 2001;31:3394–402.
[63] Kotiranta-Ainamo A, Rautonen J, Rautonen N. Imbalanced cytokine secretion in newborns. Biol Neonate 2004;85:55–60.
[64] Yu HR, Chang JC, Chen RF, et al. Different antigens trigger different Th1/Th2 reactions in neonatal mononuclear cells (MNCs) relating to T-bet/GATA-3 expression. J Leukoc Biol 2003;74:952–8.
[65] Mäkelä PH, Sibakov M, Herva E, et al. Pneumococcal vaccine and otitis media. Lancet 1980;2:547–51.
[66] Timens W, Boes A, Rozeboom-Uiterwijk T, Poppema S. Immaturity of the human splenic marginal zone in infancy: possible contribution to the deficient infant immune response. J Immunol 1989;143:3200–6.
[67] Rijkers GT, Sanders EA, Breukels MA, Zegers BJ. Infant B cell responses to polysaccharide determinants. Vaccine 1998;16:1396–400.
[68] De Rosa SC, Andrus JP, Perfetto SP, et al. Ontogeny of gamma delta T cells in humans. J Immunol 2004;172:1637–45.
[69] Gleeson M, Cripps AW. Development of mucosal immunity in the first year of life and relationship to sudden infant death syndrome. FEMS Immunol Med Microbiol 2004;42: 21–33.
[70] van Benten IJ, van Drunen CM, Koopman LP, et al. Age- and infection-related maturation of the nasal immune response in 0–2-year-old children. Allergy 2005;60:226–32.
[71] Martinez FD, Holt PG. Role of microbial burden in aetiology of allergy and asthma. Lancet 1999;354:SII12–5.
[72] Culley FJ, Pollott J, Openshaw PJ. Age at first viral infection determines the pattern of T cell-mediated disease during reinfection in adulthood. J Exp Med 2002;196:1381–6.
[73] Schwarze J, O'Donnell DR, Rohwedder A, Openshaw PJM. Latency and persistence of respiratory syncytial virus despite T cell immunity. Am J Respir Crit Care Med 2004;169: 801–5.
[74] Sims DG, Downham MA, Gardner PS, Webb JK, Weightman D. Study of 8-year-old children with a history of respiratory syncytial virus bronchiolitis in infancy. BMJ 1978;1: 11–4.
[75] Pullan CR, Hey EN. Wheezing, asthma, and pulmonary dysfunction 10 years after infection with respiratory syncytial virus in infancy. BMJ 1982;284:1665–9.
[76] Mok JY, Simpson H. Outcome of acute lower respiratory tract infection in infants: preliminary report of seven-year follow-up study. BMJ 1982;285:333–7.
[77] McConnochie KM, Roghmann KJ. Bronchiolitis as a possible cause of wheezing in childhood: new evidence. Pediatrics 1984;74:1–10.
[78] McConnochie KM, Mark JD, McBride JT, et al. Normal pulmonary function measurements and airway reactivity in childhood after mild bronchiolitis. J Pediatr 1985;107:54–8.

[79] McConnochie KM, Roghmann KJ. Wheezing at 8 and 13 years: changing importance of bronchiolitis and passive smoking. Pediatr Pulmonol 1989;6:138–46.
[80] Carlsen KH, Larsen S, Bjerve O, Leegaard J. Acute bronchiolitis: predisposing factors and characterization of infants at risk. Pediatr Pulmonol 1987;3:153–60.
[81] Osundwa VM, Dawod ST, Ehlayel M. Recurrent wheezing in children with respiratory syncytial virus (RSV) bronchiolitis in Qatar. Eur J Pediatr 1993;152:1001–3.
[82] Noble V, Murray M, Webb MS, Alexander J, Swarbrick AS, Milner AD. Respiratory status and allergy nine to 10 years after acute bronchiolitis. Arch Dis Child 1997;76:315–9.
[83] Weber MW, Milligan P, Giadom B, et al. Respiratory illness after severe respiratory syncytial virus disease in infancy in The Gambia. J Pediatr 1999;135:683–8.
[84] Kneyber MCJ, Steyerberg EW, de Groot R, Moll HA. Long-term effects of respiratory syncytial virus (RSV) bronchiolitis in infants and young children: a quantitative review. Acta Pediatr 2000;89:654–60.
[85] Piippo-Savolainen E, Remes S, Kannisto S, Korhonen K, Korppi M. Asthma and lung function 20 years after wheezing in infancy: results from a prospective follow-up study. Arch Pediatr Adolesc Med 2004;158:1070–6.
[86] Sigurs N, Bjarnason R, Sigurbergsson F, Kjellman B, Bjorksten B. Asthma and immunoglobulin E antibodies after respiratory syncytial virus bronchiolitis: a prospective cohort study with matched controls. Pediatrics 1995;95:500–5.
[87] Lehtinen P, Ruohola A, Vuorinen T, Vanto T, Jartti T, Ruuskanen O. Development of asthma after first time viral bronchiolitis [Abstract]. Presented at Frontiers in Neonatal and Infant Immunity. Madrid, Spain, March 18–20, 2005.
[88] Martinez FD, Stern DA, Wright AL, Taussig LM, Halonen M. Differential immune responses to acute lower respiratory illness in early life and subsequent development of persistent wheezing and asthma. J Allergy Clin Immunol 1998;102:915–20.
[89] Ehlenfield DR, Cameron K, Welliver RC. Eosinophilia at the time of respiratory syncytial virus bronchiolitis predicts childhood reactive airway disease. Pediatrics 2000;105:79–83.
[90] Lowe L, Murray CS, Martin L, et al. Reported versus confirmed wheeze and lung function in early life. Arch Dis Child 2004;89:540–3.
[91] Devulapalli CS, Haaland G, Pettersen M, Carlsen KH, Lodrup Carlsen KC. Effect of inhaled steroids on lung function in young children: a cohort study. Eur Respir J 2004;23: 869–75.
[92] Zambrano JC, Carper HT, Rakes GP, et al. Experimental rhinovirus challenges in adults with mild asthma: response to infection in relation to IgE. J Allergy Clin Immunol 2003; 111:1008–16.
[93] Gern JE, Calhoun W, Swenson C, Shen G, Busse WW. Rhinovirus infection preferentially increases lower airway responsiveness in allergic subjects. Am J Respir Crit Care Med 1997; 155:1872–6.
[94] Papi A, Johnston SL. Rhinovirus infection induces expression of its own receptor intercellular adhesion molecule 1 (ICAM-1) via increased NF-kappaB-mediated transcription. J Biol Chem 1999;274:9707–20.
[95] Bianco A, Sethi SK, Allen JT, Knight RA, Spiteri MA. Th2 cytokines exert a dominant influence on epithelial cell expression of the major group human rhinovirus receptor, ICAM-1. Eur Respir J 1998;12:619–26.
[96] Grunberg K, Timmers MC, Smits HH, et al. Effect of experimental rhinovirus 16 colds on airway hyperresponsiveness to histamine and interleukin-8 in nasal lavage in asthmatic subjects in vivo. Clin Exp Allergy 1997;27:36–45.
[97] Parry DE, Busse WW, Sukow KA, Dick CR, Swenson C, Gern JE. Rhinovirus-induced PBMC responses and outcome of experimental infection in allergic subjects. J Allergy Clin Immunol 2000;105:692–8.
[98] Gern JE, Vrtis R, Grindle KA, Swenson C, Busse WW. Relationship of upper and lower airway cytokines to outcome of experimental rhinovirus infection. Am J Respir Crit Care Med 2000;162:2226–31.

[99] Brooks GD, Buchta KA, Swenson CA, Gern JE, Busse WW. Rhinovirus-induced interferon-gamma and airway responsiveness in asthma. Am J Respir Crit Care Med 2003; 168:1091–4.
[100] Schwarze J, Mäkelä M, Cieslewicz G, et al. Transfer of the enhancing effect of respiratory syncytial virus infection on subsequent allergic airway sensitization by T lymphocytes. J Immunol 1999;163:5729–34.
[101] Schwarze J, Cieslewicz G, Joetham A, et al. Critical roles for interleukin-4 and interleukin-5 during respiratory syncytial virus infection in the development of airway hyperresponsiveness after airway sensitization. Am J Respir Crit Care Med 2000;162:380–6.
[102] Mäkelä MJ, Kanehiro A, Dakhama A, et al. The failure of interleukin-10-deficient mice to develop airway hyperresponsiveness is overcome by respiratory syncytial virus infection in allergen-sensitized/challenged mice. Am J Respir Crit Care Med 2002;165:824–31.
[103] Schwarze J, Gelfand EW. Respiratory viral infections as promoters of allergic sensitization and asthma in animal models. Eur Respir J 2002;19:341–9.

ELSEVIER
SAUNDERS

Infect Dis Clin N Am 19 (2005) 691–711

INFECTIOUS
DISEASE CLINICS
OF NORTH AMERICA

The Expanded Spectrum of Bartonellosis in Children

Francesco Massei, MD*, Laura Gori, MD,
Pierantonio Macchia, MD, Giuseppe Maggiore, MD

Department of Procreative Medicine and Child Development,
Division of Pediatrics, University of Pisa Hospital,
Via Roma 67, 56100 Pisa, Italy

The *Bartonella* spp are emerging infectious agents [1]. The recognition of the bacteria family Bartonellaceae has expanded in the past decade, and the genus *Bartonella* now includes 19 identified species. At least six of them (*B bacilliformis*, *B quintana*, *B henselae*, *B elizabethae*, *B vinsonii*, and *B koehlerae*) are responsible for human disease. *B henselae* represent the most frequent etiologic agent in childhood. *Bartonella* spp are small facultative fastidious intracellular gram-negative bacilli, distributed worldwide, that cause various clinical syndromes in immunocompetent and immunocompromised hosts. The term "Bartonella" takes its name from the Peruvian physician Alberto Barton, who identified *B bacilliformis*, the etiologic agent of Carrion's disease, a geographically distinct zoonosis, which was the first human disease described to be caused by a species of the genus *Bartonella*. Because the spectrum of the human disease resulting from infection with *Bartonella* spp has expanded rapidly in the past two decades, the term "bartonellosis" has been extended to a group of clinical disorders related to all major *Bartonella* species. Moreover, *Bartonella* is the only genus of bacteria capable of promoting angioproliferation through a major pathogenicity factor designated as adhesin A as observed in veruga peruana and in bacillary angiomatosis and peliosis [2]. Host immunity primarily dictates the clinical expression of the infection together with the virulence of the bacteria, the inoculation route, and the participation of vectors.

* Corresponding author.
E-mail address: f.massei@clp.med.unipi.it (F. Massei).

doi:10.1016/j.idc.2005.06.001 **id.theclinics.com**

Epidemiology

Bartonellosis has a worldwide diffusion [3]: domestic cats are the natural reservoir and vectors of *B henselae* and *B clarridgeiae*. Transmission of *B henselae* among cats is thought to occur primarily through fleas; the cat flea *Ctenocephalides felis* plays an important role in cat-to-cat transmission and a similar role may be played by ticks (*Ixodes pacificus*). Transmission from cats to humans usually occurs by a scratch or a bite and is caused by the presence of the bacterium on claws or in the oral cavity. Direct human-to-human transmission of *B henselae* infection has not been reported and there are no data supporting transmission from cats to humans by cat fleas. *Bartonella* spp can reach the claws through contact with infected flea feces present on the skin. Moreover, *Bartonella* can reach the oral cavity directly from bleeding gums or indirectly by the licking of contaminated skin [4]. Flea-infested cats tend to have higher grooming activity than noninfested cats; stray cats, cats living in a shelter, cats infected by fleas, and hunting cats are at higher risk of infection [5].

Bartonella spp infection in cats is usually asymptomatic: in experimental infection cats became bacteremic within 2 weeks after inoculation and bacteremia may persist until 32 weeks after infection [5]. Determination of the presence or absence of bacteremia is crucial in assessing the actual risk of transmission of *Bartonella* spp infection to humans; however, a non-bacteremic cat with positive serology should be re-evaluated for possible recurrent bacteremia. Feline *B henselae* isolates are genetically different and two different *B henselae* types based on partial 16S rRNA gene sequences have been described. Infection with one 16S rRNA type seems to protect from reinfection with homologous strains of *B henselae*. Whether infection with individual DNA fingerprint types of *B henselae* protects cats from infection with any other DNA fingerprint types has not been investigated. A study of cats in France showed that of 57 cats infected with *B henselae*, 41 were infected with type II, 14 were infected with type I, and 2 were coinfected with rRNA types I and II [6].

Epidemiologic studies in cats

Seroprevalence for *B henselae* varies greatly in cats and is highest in areas with warm or humid climates, which also have a higher incidence of cat flea infestation. Older cats are more likely to be seropositive and less likely to be bacteremic than younger cats. About 50% of healthy young pets at a mean age of 8 months are seropositive, and 24% of them are bacteremic [7]. Seroprevalence in cats differs considerably between different countries and between geographic regions within the same country. In North America, seroprevalence ranges in the United States from 6% in Chicago and Alaska, to 62% in California [5]; however, it is 0% in Western Canada. In Asia, a seroprevalence of 47% has been reported in Singapore [8], of 54% in

Indonesia, and of 66% in the Philippines, whereas only 15% of cats in Japan are seropositive [4]. In Australia a 35% prevalence of *B henselae* bacteremia has been reported, and in the Middle East cats' seroprevalence ranges from 40% in Israel to 12% in Egypt [4]. In European cats the higher seroprevalence was reported in The Netherlands, where 56% of domestic cats are seropositive and 22% of them bacteremic both for *B henselae* and *B clarridgeiae* [9]. In other European countries seroprevalence goes from 0% in Norway [10]; to 7% to 8.3% in Portugal [4] and in Switzerland [11], respectively; to 22.6% in Denmark [12]; to 33% in Austria; and to 41% in France [4]. In Italian cats *Bartonella* seroprevalence ranges in Central and Northern Italy from 22.9% [13] to 43% with 23% of bacteremic cats with a higher incidence of infections with *B henselae* type II, whereas the incidence of coinfection with the two genotypes is about 15% and of isolated *B clarridgiae* infection of only 5% [14].

Epidemiologic studies in humans

Seroprevalence studies of *B henselae* infection in the general population are scanty in the literature. A study in Japan reports a seroprevalence of 3.1% in patients with cardiovascular disease and of 10.9% in a high-risk population of healthy veterinarian students [15]. Two studies were performed in Greece: one in children, but with a small sample size, showing 15.9% seropositivity [16]; another on 500 healthy individuals showing 19.8% seropositivity against *B henselae* and 15% seropositivity against *B quintana* with a high percentage of cross-reactivity [17]. The authors recently performed a seroprevalence study in 508 healthy children living in Tuscany, Italy, and found 61.6% seropositivity with an IgG titer $>$1:64. Moreover, 8.4% of these children had a titer $>$1:256, currently considered indicative of recent or ongoing infection, and 3.9% of 280 IgG-positive tested sera were also positive for specific IgM [18]. Such high seroprevalence could be related to a peculiar high prevalence of this zoonosis in central Italy [13]. In the authors' study seroprevalence increased with age starting early in life supporting the hypothesis that, as the rule for many other infections in childhood, *B henselae* infection occurs in young children, is generally asymptomatic, and in most cases resolves spontaneously. This is in agreement with previous epidemiologic studies showing that almost 40% of people infected by *B quintana* during trench fever epidemics remained healthy [19] and that 60% of the inhabitants of endemic areas of Carrión's disease have a positive serology for *B bacilliformis* [19].

Clinical manifestations

The availability of a sensitive immunofluorescence assay has significantly widened in recent years the spectrum of clinical manifestations of *Bartonella* spp infections allowing the identification, particularly in childhood, of new clinical features (Box 1) [20]. Infection may occur simultaneously in siblings even with different clinical expression [21].

Cat-scratch disease

Cat-scratch disease (CSD) is the most common and typical manifestation of *B henselae* infection worldwide and consists of a subacute, solitary or regional lymphadenopathy in a patient with a previous kitten or cat contact. *B henselae* is the primary etiologic agent of CSD, but single case reports identifying *B clarridgeiae* and *B elizabethae* as the etiologic agent have been reported [22]. The clinical picture was first identified by French pediatrician Robert Debré in 1951, but attributed to *B henselae* only in 1992. The overall incidence of CSD is unknown; in the United States it is estimated in 9.3 per 100,000 population per year representing 24,000 cases annually. In the immunocompetent host, lymphadenopathy occurs 1 to 3 weeks from a scratch, bite, or other contacts with an infected kitten or cat. One or more 3- to 5-mm red-brown nontender papules develop in most patients at the site of inoculation 3 to 30 days after the infectious contact. These cutaneous lesions usually evolve through erythematous, vesicular, and papular crusted changes in 1 to 3 weeks. Affected nodes draining the site of scratch gradually enlarge, involving in order of frequency the upper extremities (46%, axillary and epitroclear nodes); the neck and jaw region (26%, cervical and submandibular nodes); the groin (17.5%, femoral and inguinal); the preauricular (7%); and the clavicular (2%) regions [23]. In 10% to 20% of cases more than one region is affected. Children are usually well-appearing with minor aspecific symptoms, such as anorexia, malaise, arthralgia, and headache. Moderate fever is present in approximately one third of patients. Lymphadenopathy is moderately tender, although some nodes are nontender. The skin over the nodes may be not inflamed, but it is often warm and erythematosus. The lymph node enlargement usually resolves within 9 weeks, but rarely lasts up to 6 to 12 months. Histologic examination reveals granulomas with multiple microabscesses. Up to 10% of lesions may suppurate requiring puncture or surgical drainage.

Because of the expanding spectrum of features related to *Bartonella* spp infection, the authors believe that the term CSD should be limited to the clinical picture of isolated lymphadenopathy. Systemic spreading of *B henselae* with organ involvement, once called atypical form of CSD, may develop independently from the presence of lymphadenopathy. Moreover, typical CSD may also precede, through a symptom-free period, systemic features of the infection [24].

Organ or tissue-specific involvement

Eye

The eye is the most common nonlymphatic affected organ in *B henselae* infection and Parinaud's oculoglandular syndrome the most common ocular complication affecting approximately 5% to 10% of patients with CSD [25]. Clinically, it is a granulomatous unilateral conjunctivitis characterized by eye redness, foreign body sensation, and serous discharge associated with preauricular lymphadenopathy. Regional lymphadenopathy may also involve submandibular or cervical nodes. Conjunctival lesions may involve the tarsal or the bulbar surface with necrosis and ulceration of the overlying epithelium. Although this syndrome can be caused by other infections including tularemia, syphilis, tuberculosis, and lymphogranuloma venereum, *B henselae* is the most frequent etiologic agent. Direct conjunctival inoculation of infected flea feces seems to be the most plausible route of infection.

Neuroretinitis is an uncommon ocular disorder presenting with an abrupt, usually unilateral, painless, visual loss. A distinctive type of retinitis referred as "Leber's" or "idiopathic stellate neuroretinitis" occurs often in children and young adults and is characterized by optic disk swelling and by a stellar macular exudate. This disorder may be isolated or may complicate a typical CDS. Recent evidence suggests that *B henselae* is the most frequent cause of stellate neuroretinitis. Some patients, however, never form a macular star, whereas other patients develop subretinal exudates and a retinochoroiditis. Pharmacologic treatment is of uncertain value; the disease is usually self-limiting in the immunocompetent host with complete recovery of vision within 3 months, but it may be rarely complicated by retinal vascular occlusion causing severe and permanent visual loss [26]. Acute intraorbital inflammation with orbital abscess deriving from an osteolitic destruction of the orbital cone has also been reported [27].

Nervous system

Acute encephalopathy is the commonest neurologic complication of *B henselae* infection [28]. After its first description in a patient with CSD in 1952, many other reports confirmed its occurrence particularly in school-age children [29]. Onset of symptoms varied from 2 days to 2 months after lymphadenopathy, when present. Progression of symptoms from headache to lethargy and coma is rapid and seizures up to status epilepticus are the predominant manifestations [30]. Less common findings described are epilepsia partialis, transient hemiplegia, acute disseminated encephalomyelitis, cerebral arteritis, aphasia, hearing loss, cranial or peripheral nerve palsy, chronic inflammatory demyelinating polyneuropathy, transverse myelitis, and meningomyeloradiculopathy [31–38]. Cerebrospinal fluid examination may be normal or may show lymphocytic pleocytosis. CT scan and MRI are usually normal or show mild, not diagnostic, changes. Treatment is mainly supportive during the acute phase because the disease is generally self-limited and usually patients recover completely without neurologic sequelae. Severe sequelae, however, such as persistent cognitive impairment and even death, has been anecdotally reported in children [39].

Box 1. Clinical manifestations of *Bartonella* spp infection in humans

Regional
  Cat-scratch disease
Disseminated with organ involvement
  Ocular
  Parinaud's oculoglandular syndrome
  Leber's stellate neuroretinitis
  Choroiditis
  Retinal detachment
  Retinal artery occlusion
  Anterior uveitis
Neurologic
  Acute encephalopathy
  Acute fatal meningoencephalitis
  Cerebritis presenting as an intracranial mass
  Cerebral arteritis
  Acute hemiplegia
  Choreoathetosis secondary to basal nerve involvement
  Status epilepticus
  Epilepsia parzialia continua
  Cerebellar ataxia
  Acute disseminated encephalomyelitis
  Persistent dementia
  Meningomyeloradiculopathy
  Demyelinating polyneuropathy
  Acute transverse myelitis
  Guillain-Barré syndrome
  Peripheral nerve paralysis (facial, palatal nerve)
Liver and gastrointestinal
  Hepatosplenic granulomatosis
  Hepatic peliosis
  Spontaneous splenic rupture
  Ileitis
  Gastrointestinal bleeding
  Abdominal lymphadenitis
  Acute gastroenteritis
  Cholestatic jaundice
Kidney
  Necrotizing glomerulonephritis
Bone
  Osteomyelitis
  Focal osteitis
  Multifocal osteitis
  Discitis

Heart and blood vessels
- Endocarditis
- Constrictive pericarditis
- Myocarditis
- Arteritis
- Henoch-Schönlein purpura
- Leukocytoclastic vasculitis

Skin
- Rashes (maculopapular petechial, morbilliform)
- Erythema nodosum
- Paronychia
- Chronic urticaria
- Cutaneous vasculitis
- Henoch-Schönlein purpura
- Erythema multiforme
- Erythema annulare
- Erythema marginatum
- Bacillary angiomatosis
- Veruga peruana

Hematologic
- Thrombocytopenia
- Autoimmune hemolytic anemia
- Nonimmune hemolytic anemia

Pleuropulmonary
- Pneumonia
- Pleural effusion
- Asymptomatic pulmonary infiltrates

Pseudoinfectious mononucleosis

Pseudomalignancy
- Histiocytosis X
- Rhabdomyosarcoma
- Breast cancer
- Inflammatory breast cancer
- Splenic lymphoma
- Parotid malignancy
- Pancreatic malignancy
- Bile duct cancer
- Cancer of the throat
- Systemic
- Oroya fever
- Trench fever
- Fever of unknown origin
- Bacillary angiomatosis
- Bacillary peliosis
- Persistent or relapsing fever with bacteremia

Liver and gastrointestinal

Visceral involvement in immunocompetent children is generally characterized by systemic symptoms, such as prolonged fever with chills, myalgia, and malaise, associated with an increase of acute phase-reactant proteins, leukocytosis, thrombocytosis, and hypergammaglobulinemia of IgG-type, and by the finding of multiple hypoechogenic-hypodense hepatic or splenic lesions (Fig. 1). Macroscopically the liver has a "nutmeg" appearance and histologic examination shows stellate necrotizing granulomata. It is noteworthy that, even in presence of severe and multiple hepatic lesions, activity of liver enzymes is always normal and hepatomegaly is rare [40]. Visceral involvement may follow a classic CSD or may develop in absence of lymphadenopathy. These patients presenting with fever of unknown origin are difficult to diagnose and in the past they have been exposed to multiple and invasive investigations. Hepatosplenic involvement even can be found in children with CDS and without systemic manifestations. Like most of the other types of organ involvement, fever and visceral lesions recover within 6 months with sometimes residual calcification. Severe abdominal pain may be present in some patients [41], sometimes as the consequence of a diffuse abdominal lymphadenitis or more rarely of a hemoperitoneum secondary to a spontaneous splenic rupture [42]. Recently, the authors investigated a child with sustained fever and increased thickness of the distal ileum on ultrasound suggesting Crohn's disease. Specific serology and the subsequent appearance of hepatosplenic lesions allowed the diagnosis of *B henselae* ileitis that resolved following a treatment with azithromycin [43]. In the spectrum of gastrointestinal manifestations of *B henselae* infection in children, acute gastroenteritis should also be considered [44].

Bone

Osteolitic lesions are often part of disseminated visceral manifestations of *B henselae* infection [24]. Lytic lesions may be observed in different sites

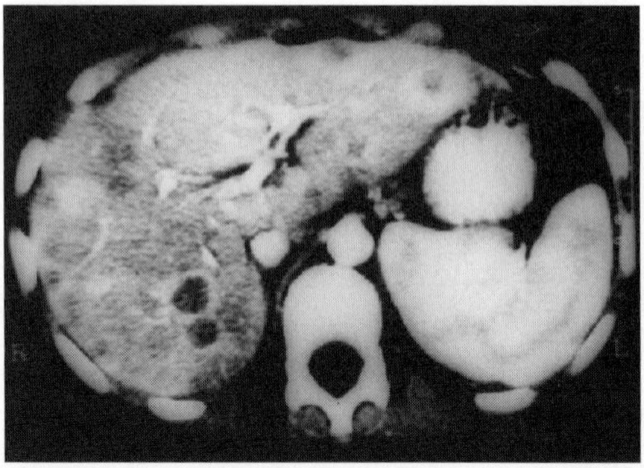

Fig. 1. Hepatosplenic involvement in disseminate *B henselae* infection. CT scan demonstrating multiple hypodense hepatic lesions.

including vertebrae, claviculae, humerus, skull, femur, sternum, acetabulum, metacarpal, and metatarsal. Bone lesions are generally distant from the inoculation site and from the enlarged nodes, but in a few cases there is a direct extension from the involved nodes to the bone [45,46]. More rarely, *B henselae* may cause a multifocal skeletal disease; in this case the differential diagnosis should include staphylococcal infection, chronic recurrent multifocal osteomyelitis, histiocytosis, and malignancy [47,48].

Heart

Five *Bartonella* spp (*B quintana*, *B henselae*, *B elizabethae*, *B vinsonii*, and *B koehlerae*) have been reported to cause different types of heart involvement (constrictive pericarditis, myocarditis, and endocarditis) [49–51]. Endocarditis is the most typical reported feature, occurring mainly in immunocompetent adults [52]. Endocarditis occurring in the absence of pre-existing valvular disease is caused prevalently by *B quintana* and is associated with distinct risk factors, such as alcoholism, homelessness, and body louse infestation. Endocarditis by *B henselae* has been reported in adults and children with previous valvular disease and with a previous contact with kitten. The evolution of the disease is insidious and the diagnosis usually delayed. Patients often present with fever, dyspnea, cardiac murmur, and acute cardiac failure. Aortic valve is often involved. Some patient may present with progressive renal insufficiency: this represents an immune complex–mediated glomerulonephritis characterized by segmental necrotizing and crescentic glomerular lesions [53]. *Bartonella* spp etiology should be considered in every patient with infectious endocarditis, negative blood cultures, and regular contact with cats. The frequency of embolic phenomena is related to the large size of the vegetations easily identified by echocardiography. Prognosis is severe, prolonged antibiotic treatment with ceftriaxone and gentamicin is required, and most patients require valve replacement.

Lung

Pleuropulmonary involvement in the form of symptomatic mono or bilateral pneumonia with pleural effusion or asymptomatic pulmonary infiltrates is rare and can be observed in systemic bartonellosis [54–56]. The presence of *B henselae* antigens in pleural fluid and in the pulmonary tissue suggests parenchymal invasion by the causative agent.

Skin

A variety of skin manifestations have been reported to occur in approximately 5% of patients with CSD. Usually these are nonspecific maculopapular rashes, but more rarely petechial, morbilliform, pruritic, or urticarial rashes and also chronic urticaria have been described [57]. In patients with systemic involvement erythema nodosum involving the pretibia and persisting for weeks or leukocytoclastic vasculitis resembling

Henoch-Schönlein purpura, suggesting a delayed hypersensitivity reaction to some bacterial antigen, have been observed [58–61]. Other skin disorders, such as erythema multiforme, erythema annulare, and erythema marginatum, have been rarely reported. The most typical cutaneous lesions related to *Bartonella* spp infection, however, are eruptive angiomatous lesions that characterize veruga peruana (caused by *B bacilliformis*) and bacillary angiomatosis. Bacillary angiomatosis is caused by *B henselae* and more rarely by *B quintana* and occurs almost exclusively in severe immunocompromised individuals, primarily in adults with acquired immunodeficiency, malignancy, or organ transplant recipients. The vasoproliferative lesions, from a few to several hundred and from a few millimeters to several centimeters, may involve the skin resembling pyogenic granuloma or may be subcutaneous. Bacillary angiomatosis can be limited to the skin and may slowly resolve spontaneously or following an appropriate antibiotic treatment, or may become disseminated [62].

Veruga peruana is an angiomatous lesion, with great histologic similarities with bacillary angiomatosis, developing in apparently immunocompetent survivors of the acute bacteremic phase of Oroya fever (see below). This systemic disorder may induce a severe $CD4^+$ lymphocyte depletion and a phagocytic dysfunction comparable with that of HIV infection.

Blood

Severe nonimmune hemolysis is the most peculiar clinical feature of Oroya fever and is caused by proliferation of *B bacilliformis* inside the erythrocytes. Severe immune-mediated thrombocytopenia and hemolytic anemia also have been described as triggered by *B henselae* infection [63,64].

Pseudomalignancy

A number of clinical conditions has been reported mostly in adults mimicking different malignancies and in particular breast cancer, when presenting with a palpable tender or nontender breast mass with axillary lymph nodes enlargement [65]; pancreatic or biliary malignancy, when presenting with an obstructive jaundice and common bile duct dilatation secondary to peripancreatic lymphadenopathy [66] or to a granulomatous mass compressing the portal vein and the biliary structures [67]; pharyngeal cancer presenting with dysphagia and a painless neck mass [68]; or a histiocytosis X when presenting with solitary osteolitic lesion of the skull [69].

Visceral angiomatous lesions often results in misdiagnosis as a malignant vascular neoplasm. They may present as an intra-abdominal mass and may produce severe life-threatening gastrointestinal bleeding eroding the intestinal wall [70]. Massive nontender lymph node enlargement in children may also suggest lymphatic malignancy and even the histologic pattern of lymph node needle biopsy may mimic lymphoma [20,71].

Pseudoinfectious mononucleosis

The clinical picture of infectious mononucleosis (fever, pharyngotonsillitis, notable cervical or submandibular lymphadenopathy, nasal obstruction, periorbital edema, and splenomegaly) may be related to various etiologies, mostly infectious (Epstein-Barr virus, cytomegalovirus, *Toxoplasma gondii*, adenovirus, rubella, HIV, and herpes viruses). This same clinical picture has been described in *B henselae* infection. Laboratory findings, however, are different from typical infectious mononucleosis because neutrophilia rather than lymphomonocytosis characterizes the blood smear of these patients. Other laboratory features include increased erythrocyte sedimentation rate and C-reactive protein, and hypergammaglobulinemia, which can be notable. Antibiotic treatment is of doubtful efficacy and all patients recover [72].

Systemic manifestations

The first described disorder related to the genus *Bartonella* was a systemic disease called Carrión's disease. This disease is endemic in an area of South America including parts of Peru, Ecuador, Bolivia, and Chile, only between the altitudes of 500 and 3200 m above sea, reflecting the habits of the sand fly vector (*Lutzomyia verrucosum*). Carrión's disease is characterized by two predominant features clinically and chronologically distinctive, but caused by the same etiologic agent, *B bacilliformis*. This organism causes a wide clinical course from a latent bacteremia to an acute fulminant and fatal illness called Oroya fever, which can be complicated some months later by an eruption of cutaneous hemangiomatous lesions called veruga peruana. Carrión's disease derives its name from a Peruvian medical student who first demonstrated the unitary etiology of the two distinct clinical pictures by inoculating himself with blood coming from a "veruga" and by developing a fatal Oroya fever. *B bacilliformis* first proliferate into the endothelial cells parasitizing subsequently the erythrocytes and causing fever and severe hemolysis. Patients who survive this acute phase may develop verrucae, which are pathognomonic of the disease.

Persistent or relapsing fever associated with myalgias, arthralgias, and bone pain (especially in the shins) and splenomegaly are the aspecific clinical features of trench fever [19], caused by *B quintana* and affecting primarily poor, homeless alcoholic men living in urban areas. The human body louse (*Pediculus humanus corporis*) is the vector and humans are the only reservoir.

Prolonged fever of unknown origin in children is of infectious origin in about 50% of the cases with an established diagnosis. In a prospective evaluation covering a 5-year period, Epstein-Barr virus infection with or without clinical mononucleosis represented the most frequent diagnosis (15%) followed by osteomyelitis of the axial skeleton (9.6%). In this series

B henselae represented the third absolute etiology accounting for 4.8% of cases [73]. Patients with fever of unknown origin have an elevated erythrocyte sedimentation rate, high C-reactive protein levels, thrombocytosis, and hypergammaglobulinemia. A history of kitten contact and the presence of visceral involvement, mainly hepatosplenic granulomatosis, are of significant diagnostic help.

Immunocompromised hosts may develop disseminated bacillary angiomatosis [62] involving brain, liver, spleen, bone marrow, and lungs. Disseminated bacillary angiomatosis is characterized by systemic symptoms including fever, chills, night sweats, anorexia, and weight loss and it may also occur in absence of pathognomonic skin lesions. Bacillary peliosis [74] occurs in terminally ill patients with acquired immunodeficiency affecting parenchymal organs with reticuloendothelial elements, primarily the liver but also involving spleen, bone marrow, and abdominal lymph nodes. It is a vasoproliferative condition where blood-filled cystic spaces are surrounded by a fibromixoid stroma in which bacteria can be identified. Incidence of bacillary angiomatosis has dramatically reduced following the introduction of AIDS tritherapy and antibiotic prophylaxis.

Persistent or relapsing fever with bacteremia is another distinct clinical feature occurring in immunocompromised individuals. All these conditions are caused by B *henselae* and *B quintana*.

Diagnosis

The diagnosis of *B henselae* infection must be suspected on anamnestic and clinical criteria, whereas laboratory tests (serology, molecular biology procedures, cultural methods, histologic investigations) allow confirmation the diagnostic suspicion. The anamnestic criterion of an intimate contact with kittens often represents a simple and useful element of suspicion; in typical CSD it is moreover essential to examine the skin for scratches, bites, and inoculation papules on the side of the adenopathy to avoid invasive procedures, such as needle biopsy.

Common laboratory tests are of limited value in suggesting *B henselae* infection: polymorphonuclear leukocytosis and evidence of increase of acute phase-reactant proteins may be evocative in disseminated disease, suggesting an abdominal ultrasound be performed for the presence multiple hypoechogenic hepatic or splenic lesions. In the past years, before the availability of a specific serology, invasive procedures were often difficult to avoid in cases of visceral involvement or of pseudomalignancy and the diagnosis of *B henselae* infection was based both on a positive skin test, currently discouraged because of the low standardization and the potential transmission of infectious agents, and on exclusion of other possible etiologies.

Serology had produced a true revolution in the diagnosis of *B henselae* infection and at present it represents the simplest laboratory procedure available to confirm the diagnosis. Indirect fluorescent antibody test and the enzyme immunoassay are the methods used for detection of specific serum antibody to *B henselae*. These tests are currently available in most laboratories and are the methods of choice to screen a patient with suspected infection. Such tests can be challenging, however, because of the different pattern of the timing of specific IgG and IgM response in single patients: some patients may produce high levels of both IgG and IgM, whereas others may produce only high levels of IgM without IgG seroconversion, and finally few patients produce only low levels of IgG and IgM classes of antibody [75].

The indirect fluorescent antibody test is the most widely used and reliable serologic test, showing 88% sensitivity and 97% specificity for IgG and IgM antibodies [76]. The variable sensitivity of different indirect fluorescent antibody tests, which are related to the antigen used, the cutoff chosen, and the test procedures used, may explain the lack of uniformity between the different serologic studies [77].

An indirect antibody IgG titer $>1:256$ is currently considered indicative of recent infection [78], even if some authors consider just a single titer $>1:64$ to be indicative of infection [79,80]. Because some patients with past disease or repeated contacts with a kitten (about 4%) may maintain a titer $>1:64$ for long periods (2–6 months), some authors [77] have proposed that one result $>1:512$ or an IgG titer increasing four dilutions in a period of 2 to 4 weeks should be required for a diagnosis of acute *B henselae* infection. The presence of specific IgM generally indicates recent or ongoing infection [81], even if false-positive results during acute Epstein-Barr virus infection have been reported [80].

There are few reports about the kinetics of anti–*B henselae* antibodies: a recent study showed that specific IgM may remain positive as long as 3 months in about 50% of the patients and in 4% for more than 3 months, whereas IgG titers usually decreased over a longer period of time, remaining positive for more than 2 years after disease onset [82]. In the same study only 25% of IgG-positive patients became seronegative 1 year after the onset of disease. Furthermore, the authors observed the absence of correlation between antibody titers, their kinetics, and the clinical spectrum of the disease.

Because of cross-reactivity between *Bartonella* spp (particularly *B henselae* and *B quintana*) and other bacteria, such as *Chlamydia psittaci*, serologic tests do not yet reliably distinguish among the different species. For this purpose the polymerase chain reaction test is considered the most sensitive available test for detecting the presence of specific DNA sequences of different species in tissues and body fluids; it is also capable of identifying distinct genotypes within the species of *Bartonella*.

Bartonella ssp can also be cultured from various tissues (blood, lymph nodes, and other tissues), but this method is diagnostically impractical for several reasons: it is slow-growing (9–40 days); there is a long period for incubation (6 weeks); and live organism is rarely isolated from blood or tissues of infected patients [83]. Although *B henselae* DNA assessment by polymerase chain reaction can be a useful tool, it can be detected in blood only in the first 6 weeks from onset, whereas most patients are currently investigated several weeks after the onset of the disease [84].

When a biopsy is available, within the granulomatous tissue it is possible to demonstrate retrospectively the bacilli within the lesions by the Warthin-Starry stain reaction (Fig. 2) or by identifying specific DNA sequences with polymerase chain reaction.

Treatment

The treatment of *B henselae* infection is different in cases of immunocompetent or immunocompromised patients. In the immunocompetent host indication for antibiotic treatment and its type and duration are controversial. Various studies have shown a significant discordance between in vitro activity of antibiotics and their clinical efficacy. Most isolates of *Bartonella* spp are indeed sensitive in vitro to many antibiotics, such as gentamicin, tetracycline, doxycycline, minocycline, erythromycin, azithromycin, clarithromycin, amoxicillin, cefotaxime, ceftriaxone, and rifampicin; and, with a variable sensitivity, to clindamycin, quinolone, and cotrimoxazole [84–87]. These antibiotics are less effective in clinical practice, however, because *Bartonella* is an intracellular bacteria [86] and poor response to penicillin derivates has been found despite apparent susceptibility in vitro. Using a cell-line assay Musso and coworkers [88] found that only aminoglycosides were bactericidal, whereas Ives and coworkers [89] found that clarithromycin, roxithromycin, and azithromycin were also efficacious in CSD.

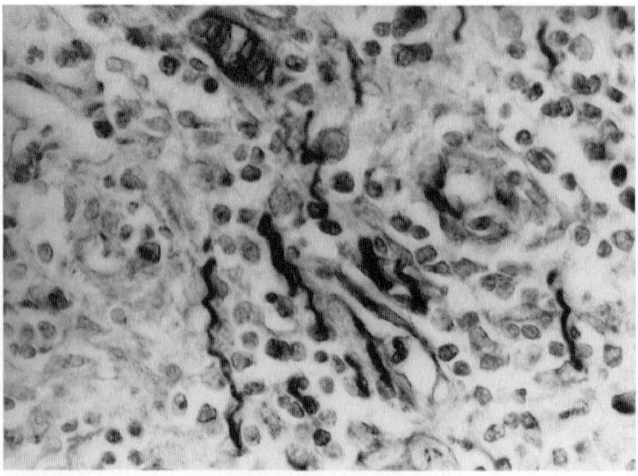

Fig. 2. Necrotizing granuloma in bone tissue. Warthin-Starry stain demonstrates pleomorphic bacilli inside the lesion.

In 1992 Margileth [90], reviewing retrospectively the effects of 18 different antibiotics in the treatment of 268 patients with typical CSD, found that only three oral antibiotics (rifampin, ciprofloxacin, and trimethoprim-sulfamethoxazole) and one parenteral (gentamicin sulfate) were efficacious. He also found that the mean duration of the illness was 14.5 weeks for patients without treatment, 14.3 weeks for patients treated with an antibiotic considered ineffective, and 2.8 weeks for patients treated with effective drugs. He concluded that antibiotic therapy should be considered for patients with severe *B henselae* infection, whereas symptomatic and conservative treatment may be recommended for most patients with mild or moderate disease.

In 1998, Chia and coworkers [91] reported a successful treatment of four patients with CSD using azithromycin administered for a 5- to 10-day course, and Bass and coworkers [92] published in the same year a prospective randomized, double-blind, placebo-controlled study on the efficacy of azithromycin for the treatment of CSD. In this study, 14 patients were treated with azithromycin and 15 were given placebo. During the first 30 days there was an 80% decrease of the initial lymph node volume in 7 of the 14 azithromycin-treated patients as compared with 1 of 15 placebo-treated controls. After 30 days there was no significant difference in the rate or the degree of resolution of the adenopathy between the two groups. The authors concluded that treatment of patients with typical CSD with oral azithromycin for 5 days affords significant clinical benefit as measured by total decrease in lymph node size but only during the first 30 days of the illness. Azithromycin penetrates both macrophages and neutrophils and is highly effective against *Bartonella* spp in a cell-free medium. The preferential concentration of azithromycin within the infected lymph node tissue and the phagocytic cells may be the reason for the drug's effectiveness against sequestered, drug-susceptible *B henselae* [91].

In children with CSD and extensive lymphadenopathy, the treatment with an azithromycin regimen consists of 10 mg/kg as a single daily dose for children weighing less than 45 kg at the first day, followed by 5 mg/kg for the following 4 days [93,94]. Because CDS is generally a self-limited disease resolving spontaneously within 1 to 3 months, most authors recommend, in immunocompetent hosts, an antibiotic treatment only in case of unresolved lymphadenopathy or when lymphadenopathy is associated with significant morbidity, or systemic disease with severe organ involvement [90,92–95], whereas for most patients treatment should be only symptomatic. Suppurative lymph nodes that become tense and extremely painful should be drained by needle aspiration. Incision and drainage of nonsuppurative nodes should be avoided because chronic draining sinuses may result. Surgical excision of the node is rarely necessary [96].

In case of systemic *B henselae* infection with hepatosplenic involvement in immunocompetent host, even if the efficacy of antimicrobial therapy is doubtful, it is reasonable to institute antibiotic therapy using one or more of the following drugs: gentamicin, trimethoprim-sulfamethoxazole, rifampin, or ciprofloxacin. A therapeutic schedule proposed by Dunn and coworkers [41] uses intravenous gentamicin (2.5 mg/kg dose every 8 hours) until apyrexia and subsequently trimethoprim-sulfamethoxazole (5 mg/kg dose every 12 hours) and rifampin (10 mg/kg dose every 12 hours) for 2 to 4 weeks. In the authors' experience azithromycin has proved to be useful in systemic forms.

In adult immunocompetent patients, various antibiotic regimens have been proposed to treat severe organ involvement, such as neuroretinitis, endocarditis, necrotizing glomerulonephritis, or encephalopathy. The combination of doxycycline (100 mg oral or intravenous twice daily) with rifampin (300 mg twice daily) has been reported successful in treating patients with neuroretinitis [93], and Reed and coworkers [97] asserted that doxycycline and rifampin seemed to shorten the course of neuroretinitis hastening the visual recovery. Experience with antimicrobial therapy in *B henselae* encephalopathy is limited to anecdotal reports: the combination of doxycycline and rifampin has been recommended in such cases.

Infective endocarditis responds to β-lactams (amoxicillin or ceftriaxone) combined with aminoglycosides (netilmicin or gentamicin) for at least 2 weeks, or β-lactams combined with other drugs (doxycycline) for 6 weeks or more. Combination with surgery is reported in at least 90% of cases [98]. The optimum duration of antibiotic therapy for immunocompetent patients with systemic *Bartonella* infection has not been determined [94].

In immunocompromised patients different studies indicate that these patients should be treated with erythromycin, erythromycin plus rifampin, or doxycycline for at least 6 weeks [99]. *Bartonellosis* in immunocompromised persons has been treated successfully with a number of antimicrobial agents, including β-lactams, ineffective in treating immunocompetent patients [94].

Bacillary angiomatosis is treated successfully with erythromycin, doxycycline, isoniazid, and rifampin. A few years ago the efficacy of macrolides, such as clarithromycin and azithromycin, was reported [100]. Failure of skin lesions to resolve in patients given ciprofloxacin or trimethoprim-sulfamethoxazole has been anecdotally reported. Patients with bacillary peliosis hepatis or relapsing bacteremia should be treated with macrolides or tetracycline preferably for 6 weeks [92,95]. In HIV patients, bacillary angiomatosis responds dramatically to various antibiotics, and HIV-infected patients require at least 6 to 8 weeks of treatment. In immunocompromised patients who relapse, treatment should be continued for 4 to 6 months, and repeated relapses should be treated indefinitely [92].

Corticosteroids have been used anecdotally with doubtful efficacy in neuroretinitis, in severe systemic disease [90], and at high-dose in a few cases of encephalopathy [101].

Summary

Bartonella spp are emerging infectious agents; in particular, *B henselae* infection occurs in early childhood, is generally asymptomatic, and in most cases revolves spontaneously. It may, however, produce a wide spectrum of clinical symptoms, the most frequent feature being the typical CSD. Disseminated atypical *B henselae* infection may follow CSD after a symptom-fee period or may present de novo; in these cases diagnosis may be difficult because clinical features may mimic a large spectrum of disorders. A careful clinical history researching an intimate contact with a kitten associated with a specific serology and an abdominal ultrasound for typical hepatosplenic involvement may allow a rapid and accurate diagnosis, reassuring the family of the child and avoiding expensive and invasive diagnostic procedures.

References

[1] Breitschwerdt EB, Kordick DL. Bartonella infection in animals: carriership, reservoir potential, pathogenicity and zoonotic potential for human infection. Clin Microbiol Rev 2000;13:428–38.

[2] Riess T, Andersson SG, Lupas A, et al. Bartonella adhesin a mediates a proangiogenic host cell response. J Exp Med 2004;200:1267–78.

[3] Karem KL, Paddaock CD, Regnery RL. *Bartonella henselae, B quintana* and *B bacilliformis*: historical pathogens of emerging significance. Microbes Infect 2000;2: 1193–205.

[4] Gurfield AN, Boulouis HJ, Chomel BB, et al. Epidemiology of *Bartonella* infection in domestic cats in France. Vet Microbiol 2001;80:185–98.

[5] Guptill L, Slater L, Wu CC, et al. Experimental infection of young specific pathogen-free cats with *B henselae*. J Infect Dis 1997;176:206–16.

[6] Heller R, Artois M, Xemar V, et al. Prevalence of *Bartonella henselae* and *Bartonella clarridgeiae* in stray cats. J Clin Microbiol 1997;35:1327–31.

[7] Guptill L, Wu CC, Hogen Esch H, et al. Prevalence, risk factors and genetic diversity of *Bartonella henselae* infection in pet cats in four region of the United States. J Clin Microbiol 2004;42:652–9.

[8] Nasirundeen AMA, Thong ML. Prevalence of *Bartonella henselae* immunoglobulins G antibodies in Singaporean cats. Pediatr Infect Dis J 1999;18:276–8.

[9] Bergmans AM, De Jong CMA, Van Amerongen G, et al. Prevalence of *Bartonella* species in domestic cats in The Netherlands. J Clin Microbiol 1997;35:2256–61.

[10] Berg K, Bevanger L, Hanssen I, et al. Low prevalence of *Bartonella henselae* infections in Norwegian domestic and feral cats. APMIS 2002;110:309–14.

[11] Glaus T, Hofmann-Lehmann R, Greene C, et al. Seroprevalence of *Bartonella henselae* infection and correlation with disease status in cats in Switzerland. J Clin Microbiol 1997; 35:2883–5.

[12] Chomel BB, Boulouis JH, Petersen H, et al. Prevalence of *Bartonella* infection in domestic cats in Denmark. Vet Res 2002;33:205–13.

[13] Ebani VV, Cerri D, Adreani E. Cat scratch disease: survey on the presence of *Bartonella henselae* among cats of Tuscany. Microbiologica 2002;25:307–13.

[14] Fabbi M, De Giuli L, Tranquillo M, et al. Prevalence of *Bartonella henselae* in Italian stray cats: evaluation of serology to assess the risk of transmission of *Bartonella* to humans. J Clin Microbiol 2004;42:264–8.

[15] Kikuchi E, Marujama S, Sakai T, et al. Serological investigation of *Bartonella henselae* infection in clinically cat scratch disease-suspected patients, patients with cardiovascular diseases and healthy veterinary students in Japan. Microbiol Immunol 2002;46:313–6.
[16] Antoniou M, Economou I, Wang X, et al. Fourteen-year sero-epidemiological study of zoonoses in a Greek village. Am J Trop Med Hyg 2002;66:80–5.
[17] Tea A, Aleyiou-Daniel S, Arvanitidou M, et al. Occurrence of *Bartonella henselae* and *Bartonella quintana* in a healthy Greek population. Am J Trop Med Hyg 2003;68: 554–6.
[18] Massei F, Messina F, Gori L, et al. High prevalence of antibodies to *Bartonella henselae* among Italian children without evidence of cat scratch disease. Clin Infect Dis 2003;38: 145–8.
[19] Bass JW, Vincent JM, Person DA. The expanding spectrum of *Bartonella* infections: I Bartonellosis and trench fever. Pediatr Infect Dis J 1997;16:2–10.
[20] Massei F, Messina F, Talini I, et al. Widening of the clinical spectrum of *Bartonella henselae* infection as recognized through serodiagnostics. Eur J Pediatr 2000;159:416–9.
[21] Gonzalez DE, Correa AG, Kaplan SL. Cat scratch disease occurring in three siblings simultaneously. Pediatr Infect Dis J 2003;22:467–8.
[22] Bass JW, Vincent JM, Person DA. The expanding spectrum of *Bartonella* infections: II Cat scratch disease. Pediatr Infect Dis J 1997;16:163–79.
[23] Carithers HA. Cat scratch disease: an overview based on a study of 1200 patients. Am J Dis Child 1985;139:1124–33.
[24] Maggiore G, Massei F, Bussani R, et al. Bone pain after lymphadenitis. Eur J Pediatr 1999; 158:165–6.
[25] Cunningham ET, Koehelr JE. Ocular bartonellosis. Am J Ophthalmol 2000;130:340–9.
[26] Ormerod LD, Dailey JP. Ocular manifestations of cat-scratch disease. Curr Opin Ophtalmol 1999;10:209–15.
[27] Wong M, Isaacs D, Dorney S. Fever, abdominal pain and an intracranial mass. Pediatr Infect Dis J 1995;14:725–8.
[28] McGrath N, Wallis W. Cat scratch encephalopathy. Neurology 1998;51:1299.
[29] Carithers HA, Margileth AM. Cat-scratch disease: acute encephalopathy and other neurological manifestations. Am J Dis Child 1991;145:98–101.
[30] Armengol EC, Hendley JO. Cat scratch disease encephalopathy: a cause of status epilepticus in school-aged children. J Pediatr 1999;134:635–8.
[31] Rocha JL, Pellegrino LN, Riella LV, et al. Acute hemiplegia associated with cat scratch disease. Braz J Infect Dis 2004;8:263–6.
[32] Walter SR, Elpes SC. Cat scratch disease presenting with peripheral facial nerve paralysis. Pediatrics 1998;101:13.
[33] Puligheddu M, Giageddu A, Genugu F, et al. Epilepsia partialis in cat scratch disease. Seizure 2004;13:191–5.
[34] Murthy SNK, Faden HS, Cohen ME, et al. Acute disseminated encephalomyelitis in children. Pediatrics 2002;110:e21.
[35] Selby G, Walker GL. Cerebral arteritis in cat scratch disease. Neurology 1979;29:1413–8.
[36] McNeil PM, Verrips A, Mullaart R, et al. Chronic inflammatory demyelinating polyneuropathy as complication of cat scratch disease. J Neurol Neurosurg Psychiatry 2000; 68:797.
[37] Salgado CD, Weisse ME. Transverse myelitis associated with probable cat-scratch disease in a previously healthy pediatric patient. Clin Infect Dis 2000;31:609–11.
[38] Hmaimess G, Kadhi H, Saint Martin C, et al. Cat scratch disease presenting as meningomyeloradiculopathy. Arch Dis Child 2004;89:691–2.
[39] Gerber JE, Jhonson JE, Schott MA, et al. Fatal meningitis and encephalitis due to *Bartonella henselae* bacteria. J Forensic Sci 2002;47:640–4.
[40] Ventura A, Massei F, Not T, et al. Systemic *Bartonella henselae* infection with hepatosplenic involvement. J Pediatr Gastroenterol Nutr 1999;29:52–6.

[41] Dunn MW, Berkowitz FE, Miller JJ, et al. Hepatosplenic cat-scratch disease and abdominal pain. Pediatr Infect Dis J 1997;16:269–72.
[42] Daybell D, Paddock CD, Zaki SR, et al. Disseminated infection with *Bartonella henselae* as a cause of spontaneous splenic rupture. Clin Infect Dis 2004;39:e21–4.
[43] Massei F, Massimetti M, Messina F, et al. *Bartonella henselae* and inflammatory bowel disease. Lancet 2000;356:1245–6.
[44] Liapi-Adamidou G, Tsolia M, Magiakou AM, et al. Cat scratch disease in 2 siblings presenting as acute gastroenteritis. Scand J Infect Dis 2000;32:317–9.
[45] Carithers HA. Cat-scratch disease associated with an osteolytic lesion. Am J Dis Child 1983;137:968–70.
[46] Shanon ABZ, Marchessault JHV. Cat-scratch disease associated with a vertebral osteolytic lesion. Pediatr Inf Dis J 1989;8:51–2.
[47] Gallemore G, Worley K. Cat scratch disease presenting as multifocal osteitis. Tenn Med 1996;89:289–90.
[48] Modi SP, Epps SC, Klei JD. Cat scratch disease presenting as multifocal osteomyelitis with thoracic abscess. Pediatr Infect Dis 2001;20:1006–7.
[49] Baorto E, Payne RM, Slater L, et al. Culture-negative endocarditis caused by *Bartonella*. J Pediatr 1998;132:1051–4.
[50] Bharti DR, Mehta AV. Constrictive pericarditis following cat-scratch disease in a 12-year-old female: a rare association. Tenn Med 2003;96:509–10.
[51] Meininger GR, Nadasdy T, Hruban RH, et al. Chronic active myocarditis following acute *Bartonella henselae* infection (cat scratch disease). Am J Surg Pathol 2001;25:1211–4.
[52] Broukui P, Raoult D. Endocarditis due to rare and fastidious bacteria. Clin Microbiol Rev 2001;14:177–207.
[53] Bookman I, Scholey JW, Jassal SW, et al. Necrotizing glomerulonephritis secondary to *Bartonella henselae* endocarditis. Am J Kidney Dis 2004;43:25–30.
[54] Margileth AM, Baehren DF. Chest-wall abscess due to cat-scratch disease in an adult with antibodies to *Bartonella clarridgeiae*: case report and review of the thoracopulmonary manifestations of CSD. Clin Infect Dis 1998;27:353–7.
[55] Abbasi S, Chesney PJ. Pulmonary manifestations of cat-scratch disease: a case report and review of the literature. Pediatr Infect Dis J 1995;14:547–8.
[56] Marseglia GL, Monafo V, Marone P, et al. Asymptomatic persistent pulmonary infiltrates in an immunocompetent boy with cat-scratch disease. Eur J Pediatr 2001;160:260–5.
[57] Chian CA, Arrese JE, Piérard GE. Skin manifestation of *Bartonella* infections. Int J Dermatol 2002;41:461–6.
[58] Sander A, Frank B. Paronychia caused by *Bartonella henselae*. Lancet 1997;350:1078.
[59] Sundaresh KV, Madjar DD Jr, Camisa C, et al. Cat scratch disease associated with erythema nodosum. Cutis 1986;38:317–9.
[60] Ayoub EM, McBride J, Schmiederer M, et al. Role of *Bartonella henselae* in the etiology of Henoch-Schönlein purpura. Pediatr Infect Dis J 2002;21:28–31.
[61] Hashkes PJ, Trabulsi A, Passo MH. Systemic cat-scratch disease presenting as leukocytoclastic vasculitis. Pediatr Infect Dis J 1996;15:93–5.
[62] Adal KA, Cockerell CJ, Petri WA. Cat-scratch disease, bacillary angiomatosis and other infections due to Rochalimaea. N Engl J Med 1994;330:1509–15.
[63] Borker A, Gadner R. Severe thrombocytopenic purpura as a complication of cat scratch disease. Clin Pediatr 2002;41:117–8.
[64] Van Audenhove A, Verhoff G, et al. Autoimmune haemolytic anaemia triggered by *Bartonella henselae* infection: a case report. Br J Haematol 2001;115:924–5.
[65] Markaki S, Sotiropoulou M, Papaspirou P, et al. Cat-scratch disease presenting as a solitary tumour in the breast: report of three cases. Eur J Obstet Gynecol Reprod Biol 2003;106:175–6.
[66] Raasveld MHM, Weel JFL, Braat MCP, et al. Cat-scratch disease mimicking pancreatic malignancy: case report. Clin Infect Dis 1997;24:77–8.

[67] Zinzindohoue F, Guiard-Schmid JB, La Scola B, et al. Portal triad involvement in cat-scratch disease. Lancet 1996;348:1178–9.
[68] Ridder GJ, Richet B, Laszing R, et al. A farmer with a lump in his throat. Lancet 1998;351: 954.
[69] Berg LC, Norelle A, Morgan WA, et al. Cat-scratch disease simulating histiocytosis X. Hum Pathol 1998;29:649–51.
[70] Koehler JE, Cederberg L. Intra-abdominal mass associated with gastrointestinal hemorrhage: a new manifestation of bacillary angiomatosis. Gastroenterology 1995;109: 2011–4.
[71] Ghez D, Bernard L, Bayou E, et al. *Bartonella henselae* infection mimicking a splenic lymphoma. Scand J Infect Dis 2001;33:935–6.
[72] Massei F, Messina F, Massimetti M, et al. Pseudoinfectious mononucleosis: a presentation of *Bartonella henselae* infection. Arch Dis Child 2000;83:443–4.
[73] Jacobs JR, Schutze GE. *Bartonella henselae* as a cause of prolonged fever and fever of unknown origin in children. Clin Infect Dis 1998;26:80–4.
[74] Perkocha LA, Geaghan SM, Benedict TS. Clinical and pathological features of bacillary peliosis hepatis in association with human immunodeficiency virus infection. N Engl J Med 1990;323:1581–6.
[75] Bergmans AM, Peeters MF, Schellekens JF, et al. Pitfalls and fallacies of cat scratch disease serology: evaluation of *Bartonella henselae*-based indirect fluorescence assay and enzyme-linked immunoassay. J Clin Microbiol 1997;35:1931–7.
[76] Sherreen B, Demers DM. Spectrum and treatment of cat scratch disease. Pediatr Infect Dis J 2004;23:1161–2.
[77] Sander A, Berner R, Ruess M. Serodiagnosis of cat scratch disease: response to *Bartonella henselae* in children and review of diagnostic methods. Eur J Clin Microbiol Infect Dis 2001; 20:392–401.
[78] Nadal D, Zbinden R. Serology to *Bartonella (Rochalimaea) henselae*, may replace traditional diagnostic criteria for cat scratch disease. Eur J Pediatr 1995;154:906–8.
[79] Karpathios T, Golphinos C, Psycou P, et al. Cat scratch disease in Greece. Arch Dis Child 1998;78:64–6.
[80] Zbinden R, Strohle A, Nadal D. IgM to *Bartonella henselae* in cat scratch disease during acute Epstein Barr virus infection. Med Microbiol Immunol 1998;186:167–70.
[81] Not T, Canciani M, Buratti E, et al. Serologic response to *Bartonella henselae* in patients with cat scratch disease and in sick and in healthy children. Acta Paediatr 1999;88:1–6.
[82] Metzkor-Cotter E, Kletter Y, Avidor B, et al. Long-term serological analysis and clinical follow-up of patients with cat scratch disease. Clin Infect Dis 2003;37:1149–54.
[83] Dalton MJ, Olson JG. Bartonella species (cat scratch disease, bacillary angiomatosis). In: Long SS, Pickering LK, Prober CG, editors. Principles and practice of pediatric infectious diseases. 1st edition. New York: Churchill Livingstone; 1997. p. 968–72.
[84] Manfredi R, Sabbatani S, Chiodo F. Bartonellosis: light and shadows in diagnostic and therapeutic issues. Clin Microbiol Infect 2005;11:167–9.
[85] Maurin M, Raoult D. Antimicrobial susceptibility of *Rochalimaea quintana*, *Rochalimaea vinsonii* and the newly recognized *Rochalimaea henselae*. J Antimicrob Chemother 1993;32: 587–94.
[86] Windsor JJ. Cat-scratch disease: epidemiology, aetiology and treatment. Br J Biomed Sci 2001;58:101–10.
[87] Greub G, Raoult D. Bartonella: new explanations for old disease. J Med Microbiol 2002; 51:915–23.
[88] Musso D, Drancourt M, Raoult D. Lack of bactericidal effect of antibiotics expect aminoglycosides on *Bartonella (Rochalimaea) henselae*. J Antimicrob Chemother 1995;36: 101–8.
[89] Ives TJ, Manzewitsch P, Regnery RL, et al. In vitro susceptibilities of *Bartonella henselae*, *B quintana*, *B elizabethae*, *Rickettsia rickettsii*, *R. conorii*, *R. akari* and *R. prowazekii* to

macrolide antibiotics as determined by immunofluorescent-antibody analysis of infected vero cell monolayers. Antimicrob Agents Chemother 1997;41:578–82.
[90] Margileth AM. Antibiotic therapy for cat-scratch disease: clinical study of therapeutic outcome in 268 patients and a review of the literature. Pediatr Infect Dis J 1992;11:474–8.
[91] Chia JKS, Nakata MM, Lami JLM, et al. Azithromycin for the treatment of cat-scratch disease. Clin Infect Dis 1998;26:193–4.
[92] Bass JW, Freitas BC, Freitas AD, et al. Prospective randomised double blind placebo-controlled evaluation of azithromycin for treatment of cat-scratch disease. Pediatr Infect Dis J 1998;17:447–52.
[93] Rolain JM, Brouqui P, Koehler JE, et al. Recommendations for treatment of human infections caused by *Bartonella* species. Antimicrob Agents Chemother 2004;48:1921–33.
[94] Conrad DA. Treatment of cat-scratch disease. Curr Opin Pediatr 2001;13:56–9.
[95] Zangwill KM. Bartonella infections. Semin Paediatr Infect Dis 1997;8:57–63.
[96] Stechenberg BW. Bartonella. In: Berhman RE, Kliegman RM, Jenson HB, editors. Textbook of pediatrics. 17th edition. Philadelphia: WB Saunders; 2004. p. 943–6.
[97] Reed JB, Scales DK, Wong MT. Bartonella henselae neuroretinitis in cat scratch disease: diagnosis, management and sequelae. Ophthalmology 1998;105:459–66.
[98] Moreillon P, Qua YA. Infective endocarditis. Lancet 2004;363:139–49.
[99] Schutze GE. Diagnosis and treatment of *Bartonella henselae* infection. Pediatr Infect Dis J 2000;19:1185–7.
[100] Guerra LG, Neira CJ, Boman G, et al. Rapid response of AIDS-related bacillary angiomatosis to azithromycin. Clin Infect Dis 1993;17:264–6.
[101] Weston KD, Tran T, Kimmel KN, et al. Possible role of high-dose corticosteroids in the treatment of cat-scratch disease encephalopathy. J Clin Neurol 2001;16:762–3.

ELSEVIER
SAUNDERS

Infect Dis Clin N Am 19 (2005) 713–729

INFECTIOUS
DISEASE CLINICS
OF NORTH AMERICA

Antiretroviral Therapy in HIV-Infected Children: The Metabolic Cost of Improved Survival

Ethan G. Leonard, MD[a,b],
Grace A. McComsey, MD[a,b,*]

[a]*Department of Pediatrics, Case Western Reserve University School of Medicine, Cleveland, OH 4410, USA*
[b]*Division of Pediatric Infectious Diseases and Rheumatology, Rainbow Babies and Children's Hospital, 11100 Euclid Avenue, Mail Stop 6008a, Cleveland, OH 4410, USA*

Tolerability of highly active antiretroviral therapy in children

The advent of highly active antiretroviral therapy (HAART) in 1996 has led to substantial declines in mortality from HIV infection in industrialized countries [1,2]. Several pediatric studies showed substantial decreases in mortality in HIV-infected children and adolescents treated with HAART [3–5]. Gortmaker et al [3] reported a decrease in mortality from 5.3% to 0.7% between 1996 and 1999 in HIV-infected children that correlated with a 10-fold increase in the usage of protease inhibitors (PIs).

The use of antiretroviral therapy (ART) in HIV-infected children has not been without complications. This article discusses the commonly encountered adverse effects of ART that may lead to noncompliance or the need to alter therapy. Most of the discussion focuses on the metabolic complications of HAART in pediatric patients and the anticipated morbidity resulting from longer survival and exposure to these therapies.

Although the adult literature is replete with studies and reviews of lipodystrophy syndrome, dyslipidemia, insulin resistance, osteopenia, and mitochondrial dysfunction in patients receiving HAART, the pediatric

Dr. McComsey serves on the Advisory Board for GlaxoSmithKline and Bristol-Myers-Squibb, but no funding was requested or received for this article.

* Corresponding author. Division of Pediatric Infectious Diseases and Rheumatology, Rainbow Babies and Children's Hospital, 11100 Euclid Avenue, Mail Stop 6008a, Cleveland, OH 44106, USA.

E-mail address: mccomsey.grace@clevelandactu.org (G.A. McComsey).

0891-5520/05/$ - see front matter
doi:10.1016/j.idc.2005.05.006 *id.theclinics.com*

literature is relatively sparse [6,7]. Not enough data exist about the long-term consequences of these metabolic derangements in children receiving HAART; however, the likely long-term exposure to these drugs makes these derangements a serious concern.

Lipodystrophy and cardiovascular disease

The lipodystrophy syndrome encompasses changes in body fat composition. The phenotypic presentation of this syndrome can be that of lipohypertrophy (accumulation of central fat), lipoatrophy (peripheral fat loss), or mixed. Studies have proposed that lipoatrophy and lipohypertrophy are frequently comorbid, but distinct entities in HIV-infected patients. Lipoatrophy is the more specific feature of fat maldistribution in HIV [8,9]. Even subjects without clinically recognized lipoatrophy had significantly less fat in the limbs on CT scan or MRI compared with age-matched, non–HIV-infected persons. The implication is that lipoatrophy is more common than initially thought, and that many HIV-infected people may have long-term "subclinical" lipoatrophy before it becomes clinically evident to physicians. Regardless of the phenotypic presentation of lipodystrophy, objective measurements remain the ideal way to establish the diagnosis and monitor subjects. The various advantages and disadvantages of commonly used techniques to assess body fat are summarized in Table 1 [7]. The entire spectrum of morphologic derangements reported in adults has been described in HIV-infected pediatric patients [10–16]. Estimates of the prevalence of clinically evident lipodystrophy syndrome in HIV-infected children range from 1% to 43% [13].

At first, PI therapy was implicated as the most likely cause of fat maldistribution [17], but more recent studies have shifted the focus to nucleoside reverse transcriptase inhibitors (NRTIs) as the primary culprit, particularly in lipoatrophy [18–20]. Lipoatrophy is uncommon in patients who are treated with NRTI-sparing regimens [21,22]. Stavudine has been overwhelmingly the most implicated NRTI [18–20,23–27]. Further data suggesting the culpability of NRTI but not PI therapy for lipoatrophy comes from the numerous therapy-switch studies. The replacement of a PI with either a non-nucleoside reverse transcriptase inhibitor or abacavir in a virologically successful regimen did not lead to improvement of the fat abnormalities despite improvements in metabolic derangements in adult and pediatric HIV-infected patients [28–31]. In contrast, therapy-switch studies to NRTI-sparing regimens [32] and changing certain NRTIs (eg, replacing stavudine with abacavir) did lead to improvement of lipoatrophy [30,33,34].

In adults, visceral adiposity is an independent risk factor for cardiovascular disease and negatively affects two other known risk factors: insulin resistance and dyslipidemia [35–41]. Hadigan et al [42] reported an increased risk of cardiovascular disease in HIV-infected patients with fat maldis-

Table 1
Advantages and disadvantages of available modalities for assessing fat maldistribution

Technique	Advantages	Disadvantages
Anthropometric measurements	Noninvasive and inexpensive modality to measure subcutaneous fat	Requires standardization and experience Does not measure visceral fat or assess regional fat distribution
Bioelectrical impedance	Noninvasive and inexpensive technique to measure lean body mass and total body fat	Does not assess regional fat distribution
DEXA	Useful tool for assessing regional fat distribution	Does not measure facial or visceral fat Minimal radiation exposure
Abdominal CT	Discriminates accurately between subcutaneous and visceral fat Rapid test Requires only a single slice for assessment of fat	Expensive Requires more radiation exposure than DEXA
MRI	Sensitive tool to measure regional fat distribution Discriminates accurately between subcutaneous and vixceral fat No radiation	Most expensive technique A long procedure that may necessitate sedation in younger patients

Abbreviation: DEXA, dual energy x-ray absorptiometry.

tribution compared with HIV-infected patients without lipodystrophy and with healthy controls. Central obesity, hyperlipidemia, and insulin resistance also are thought to be risk factors for development of cardiovascular disease in children [43–46].

Several studies have examined the relationship between HAART and cardiovascular disease in HIV-infected adults. Although Bozzette et al [47] published a large retrospective study showing no increase in cardiovascular or cerebrovascular hospitalizations in HIV-infected patients treated at Department of Veterans Affairs hospitals between 1993 and 2001, several other studies reported an increased incidence of cardiovascular disease in this population. Among these, the Data Collection on Adverse Events of Anti-HIV Drugs, a large prospective observational study, showed that combination ART was independently associated with a 26% relative increase in the rate of myocardial infarction per year of exposure during the first 4 to 5 years of use [48,49]. Mary-Krause et al [50] reported an increased rate of myocardial infarction in HIV-infected adults specifically related to duration of PI therapy.

Given the suggestion that the risk of cardiovascular disease is related to the duration of HAART therapy in adults [46,48–50], and that fat maldistribution in children is proportional to the duration of exposure to HAART [15], one might surmise that children treated with HAART would be at exceptionally high risk for premature cardiovascular morbidity and mortality. The validity of this hypothesis will soon be known, as the first generation of children to receive HAART enter their second decade. In addition to contributing to increased risk of cardiovascular disease, lipodystrophy clearly contributes to low self-esteem, depression, sexual difficulties, and potentially noncompliance with HAART therapy [51,52]. This emotional adverse event poses a particular problem for clinicians treating adolescent patients, who tend to have heightened sensitivity to body image and an age-related tendency toward noncompliance with long-term medical therapy [16].

Management strategies for lipodystrophy

Aside from the aforementioned switch strategies to NRTI-sparing regimens or replacing stavudine with abacavir, few well-studied options for improving fat maldistribution exist. Lipoatrophy has been linked to increased oxidative stress [53]. A pilot trial of antioxidant therapy in HIV-infected adults resulted in decreased waist-to-hip ratios, but not other anthropometric measurements [54]. Initially, small studies showed a potential increase in fat gain with rosiglitazone therapy in patients with HIV-associated lipoatrophy [55,56]; however, this effect was not shown in larger, randomized controlled trials [57,58]. Impaired growth hormone secretion has been associated with visceral adiposity in adults and adolescents with HIV infection [59,60]. Kotler et al [61] suggested that maintenance therapy with low-dose recombinant human growth hormone reduced visceral adipose tissue without creating insulin resistance in a group of HIV-infected adults; however, several patients did develop insulin resistance with higher dose regimens [62]. The efficacy, safety, and dosing for rosiglitazone and recombinant human growth hormone have not been determined for prepubertal HIV-infected children with lipodystrophy.

Dyslipidemia

Disorders of lipid metabolism were observed in HIV-infected adults before the advent of HAART [63]. As PI therapy became more common, the prevalence and severity of dyslipidemia increased substantially. Numerous studies implicate PI therapy with substantial increases in low-density lipoprotein cholesterol and even greater increases in serum triglyceride levels [17,64–68]. The best evidence for a direct effect of PI on lipid metabolism comes from studies of seronegative volunteers who developed dyslipidemia after a short course of PI therapy [69,70]. In one of the largest adult cohort studies, 49% of 581 HIV-infected patients had dyslipidemia as determined by fasting lipids: 33% had cholesterol greater than 212 mg/dL, 12% had high-density lipoprotein less than 35 mg/dL, 25% had triglycerides greater than 195 mg/dL, and 16% had elevations in total cholesterol and triglyceride levels [64].

Fewer data exist about the prevalence of dyslipidemia in HIV-infected children. Several small cross-sectional studies report the prevalence of elevated cholesterol to range from 13% to 75% [10,13,14,71–73]. In the largest reported cohort study of dyslipidemia in HIV-infected children, Farley et al [72] prospectively followed nearly 2000 perinatally infected children between the ages of 4 and 19 years. Approximately 13% had total cholesterol levels higher than the 95th percentile of the gender-specific, race-specific, and age-specific standards defined by the Third National Health and Nutrition Examination Survey [74]. As in the adult studies, PIs were the most implicated drug class in association with dyslipidemia in HIV-infected children. The reported prevalence of PI-induced dyslipidemia ranges from 20% of children on a single PI to greater than 90% of children being treated with regimens containing two or more PIs [10,75,76]. To date, ritonavir and nelfinavir are the two best studied PIs in children. In a small Swiss study, Chesaux et al [77] showed that although both of these drugs led to increased cholesterol levels, the children receiving ritonavir had significantly higher cholesterol and triglyceride levels compared with baseline and the nelfinavir group.

Although longitudinal data for the consequences of dyslipidemia are lacking in the pediatric population, the hypothesized consequence is the premature development of atherosclerotic disease. Chesaux et al [77] reported that HIV-infected children receiving HAART have elevations in their cholesterol similar to that seen in patients heterozygous for familial hypercholesterolemia. In the Bogalusa Heart Study, 93 autopsies were performed on subjects age 2 to 39 years, most of whom died from trauma and had antemortem data about cardiovascular risk factors [44]. The presence of fatty streaks or fibrous plaques in the coronary arteries and aorta were significantly correlated with high body mass index and cholesterol, triglyceride, and low-density lipoprotein levels. This risk for atherosclerotic diseases in a young population is quite concerning for patients in their first decade of life with lipodystrophy and dyslipidemia from ART.

Management strategies for dyslipidemia

There are currently no published data regarding the pharmacologic treatment of HIV-infected children with hyperlipidemia. The Cardiovascular Subcommittee of the AIDS Clinical Trials Group (ACTG) has suggested following the National Cholesterol Education Program guidelines for the evaluation and treatment of dyslipidemia [78,79]. The standard lipid-lowering agents, 3-hydroxy-3-methylglutaryl coenzyme A reductase inhibitors or "statins," should be used cautiously because of their metabolism by the cytochrome P-450 enzyme CYP3A4 in the liver and consequently the potential for significant drug interactions when used with PIs. In this regard, several reports of hepatitis, rhabdomyolysis, and lactic acidosis have emerged as the result of concomitant use of statins and PI therapy [80,81]. In 2002, lovastatin became the first and only of this drug class approved by the US Food and Drug Administration for the treatment of hyperlipidemia in adolescents with familial hypercholesterolemia [82]. No long-term safety data in children exist. The American Academy of Pediatrics has guidelines for the use of the acid-binding resins cholestyramine and colestipol in children older than age 10 with hyperlipidemia and at least two other cardiac risk factors [83]. These compounds may cause elevations in triglyceride levels in patients treated with PIs [81] and may interfere with antiretroviral absorption, leading to virologic failure. The fibric acid derivatives gemfibrozil and fenofibrate do lower triglyceride levels and increase HDL. The ACTG group recommends reserving therapy for patients who have triglyceride levels greater than 500 mg/dL. These drugs are metabolized by hepatic enzymes that are induced by the most commonly prescribed pediatric PIs, ritonavir and nelfinavir, and may have minimal efficacy in PI-associated dyslipidemia in HIV-infected children.

Several adult studies show that switching a patient to a PI-sparing regimen ameliorates the lipid abnormalities [30,84,85]. McComsey et al [28] have published the only pediatric PI switch study. Seventeen children receiving HAART had efavirenz substituted for their PI. After 48 weeks, they showed improvement in cholesterol, low-density lipoprotein, and triglyceride levels and loss of virologic control. There are no data to support treatment interruption in HIV-infected children. The use of PI-sparing regimens or the development of safer PIs is crucial to prevent cardiovascular morbidity for HIV-infected children. In HIV-infected adults, the new PI atazanavir has not been associated with significant elevations in lipid levels. An ongoing pediatric study will clarify if the use of this agent also will be safe and effective in children.

Insulin resistance

The Food and Drug Administration first reported an association between PI therapy and diabetes mellitus in 1997 [86]. The true prevalence of insulin resistance is difficult to determine because of a lack of standardized definitions. Given the impracticality of performing the "gold standard" measure of resistance, the euglycemic clamp, many investigators have adopted alternative, less optimal diagnostic strategies, including levels of fasting glucose, glucose after oral challenge, fasting insulin, C-peptide, and a variety of other indices such as homeostasis model assessment of insulin resistance (HOMA-IR) [18,64,87]. In HIV-infected adults, PI therapy has been implicated in the generation of insulin resistance [65,68,88,89]. In vitro, some PIs directly inhibit the insulin-stimulated glucose transport by the isoform transporter Glut-4 [90,91]. Other studies have shown hyperinsulinemia resulting from treatment with NRTIs [92,93]. The development of insulin resistance in these adults seems to be multifactorial. Body habitus, particularly increased visceral-to-subcutaneous fat ratios, has been reported to predict independently the development of insulin resistance in HIV-infected adults [94,95].

Hyperinsulinemia and hyperglycemia have been reported in HIV-infected children receiving HAART. As in their adult counterparts, children with fat maldistribution are more likely to show insulin resistance; however, the presence of numerous confounding variables precludes definitive linkage of these conditions. Bitnun et al [11], in the largest published cohort of glucose homeostasis in HIV-infected children, reported that only advanced Tanner stage correlated with insulin resistance. These authors speculated that the PI association with insulin resistance was not seen in prepubertal children in their study because of known association between prepubertal heightened insulin sensitivity and increased subcutaneous-to-visceral fat ratios [96,97].

At this point, the necessity to monitor or to treat the disordered glucose metabolism in either adult or pediatric patients is unclear. As noted earlier, insulin resistance is a known contributor to cardiovascular disease in adults regardless of HIV status. The American Heart Association and the American Diabetes Association have cited insulin resistance in a child as a major risk factor for cardiovascular disease and urge "aggressive" therapy [46].

Management strategies for insulin resistance

As for dyslipidemia, exercise and dietary modification are considered the first interventions. Hadigan et al [98] reported that insulin resistance in HIV-infected adults is significantly correlated with polyunsaturated-to-saturated fat levels and inversely with dietary fiber intake. A small French study suggested that light anaerobic exercise, although it improved lipid profiles and fat maldistribution in HIV-infected adults, did not alter derangements in glucose homeostasis [99]. In several small studies, metformin has improved glucose homeostasis in HIV-infected adults, but can result in lactic acidosis [100–102]. In the United States, the drug is licensed for use in children older than 10 years with type 2 diabetes. The thiazolidenediones, a drug class that reduces hepatic insulin resistance and increases peripheral glucose uptake, have efficacy in adult patients with type 2 diabetes [103,104]. Thiazolidenediones seem to be effective in improving insulin resistance in HIV-infected adults [56]. In HIV-infected adults, switching to a PI-sparing regimen was noted to improve insulin resistance, but the previously mentioned pediatric trial showed no significant impact of substituting efavirenz for a PI on C-peptide, insulin, or glucose levels during a 48-week study period [28,29,84]. There are currently no formal recommendations to employ switch strategies in HIV-infected adults with derangements in glucose homeostasis.

Bone disease

Bone disease in HIV-infected patients is generally divided into two categories, decreased bone mineral density (BMD) and avascular necrosis. Adults and children with HIV infection have an increased risk of avascular necrosis of the hip relative to the general population [105,106]. No evidence links avascular necrosis to ART [7,107–109].

Many studies of HIV-infected adults suggest that HIV disease itself rather than ART negatively affects bony metabolism [110–112]; even less is known about the impact of ART on children's BMD. Most studies are cross-sectional and predominantly involve HIV-infected adults, and in most cases, the study patients already had been on combination ART. The first reported study of long-term longitudinal bone assessment of HIV-infected adults revealed that osteopenia already was statistically more common in these patients before ART compared with the general population [113].

Several studies of BMD in HIV-infected children reveal significant levels of osteopenia and osteoporosis as defined by a score of dual energy x-ray absorptiometry (DEXA) less than or equal to 1 to 2 SDs below age-adjusted, gender-adjusted, and ethnic-adjusted norms [114,115]. McComsey and Leonard [115] performed DEXA evaluations on 23 vertically infected children; 26% met criteria for osteopenia, and 48% had osteoporosis. The process is insidious; none of the patients was symptomatic. These finding are quite concerning because BMD normally increases during childhood and adolescence, peaks in young adult life, and declines at a rate of approximately 0.5% to 1% per year [116]. A child who fails to reach physiologically appropriate peak bone mass would be at accelerated risk of osteoporotic fractures as the normal decline with age begins in young adulthood.

Management strategies for bone disease

Currently, DEXA testing is not recommended routinely for HIV-infected patients. Data about management of bone loss in these patients are sparse. Oxandrolone, a synthetic anabolic steroid, and recombinant human growth hormone do not improve BMD in HIV-infected adults [117,118]. A trial of vitamin D and calcium supplementation showed no improvement in DEXA score or BMD [115] of HIV-infected children. Two pilot trials of alendronate, a bisphosphonate, given for 48 weeks to HIV-infected adults with osteopenia or osteoporosis yielded modest increases in lumbar spine BMD, but the therapy was well tolerated [119,120]. A larger ongoing ACTG study will better assess the efficacy and safety of alendronate in HIV-infected adults with significantly decreased BMD. Even outside of HIV, limited data exist about the use of bisphosphonates in children, and no data about the long-term impact of this therapy on growing children exist.

Mitochondrial toxicity

Lactic acidosis frequently associated with hepatic steatosis is the extreme manifestation of NRTI-induced mitochondrial toxicity and has been reported in HIV-infected patients since the early 1990s [121,122]. Functional and structural defects in mitochondria have been shown in adults with symptomatic hyperlactatemia [123,124]. Severe lactic acidosis is rare, and symptomatic acidemia is uncommon. Observational studies suggest the incidence of severe symptoms and mild disease as 1.3 to 1.7/1000 person-years and 26/1000 person-years of NRTI exposure [123,125–127]. When patients have symptomatic lactic academia, they complain of nausea, emesis, abdominal pain, extreme fatigue, myalgia, tachycardia, dyspnea on exertion, and weight loss. Several reports of clinically significant hyperlactatemia resulting from in utero exposure to NRTI appear in the literature [128–130]. Other studies show mild elevations of serum lactate levels in infants exposed to, but ultimately found to be uninfected with, HIV when treated with NRTI therapy [131]; the elevations were transient and resolved after therapy was discontinued. The prevalence of asymptomatic hyperlactatemia has been reported to range from 6% to 36% in adults receiving NRTI therapy depending on the definition of elevated venous lactate levels [123,132,133]. In the two largest pediatric cohort studies of serum lactate, 29% to 32% of HIV-infected children had hyperlactatemia [134,135]. None of the patients had symptoms. As found in HIV-infected adults, the clinical importance of asymptomatic hyperlactatemia is unclear [133]. There are no recommendations for routine measurements of serum lactate levels in adults or children.

If a patient presents with moderate-to-severe symptoms, ART should be transiently discontinued. If possible, an NRTI-sparing regimen should be implemented. Studies suggest the potential for using NRTI drugs with less mitochondrial toxicity, such as abacavir, lamivudine, or tenofovir [136–138]. Trials with uridine supplementation for reversing mitochondrial toxicity are under way.

References

[1] Report on the global AIDS epidemic Geneva: Joint United Nations Programme on HIV/AIDS; 2004.

[2] Palella FJ Jr, Delaney KM, Moorman AC, et al. Declining morbidity and mortality among patients with advanced human immunodeficiency virus infection. HIV Outpatient Study Investigators. N Engl J Med 1998;338:853.

[3] Gortmaker SL, Hughes M, Cervia J, et al. Effect of combination therapy including protease inhibitors on mortality among children and adolescents infected with HIV-1. N Engl J Med 2001;345:1522.

[4] Viani RM, Araneta MR, Deville JG, Spector SA. Decrease in hospitalization and mortality rates among children with perinatally acquired HIV type 1 infection receiving highly active antiretroviral therapy. Clin Infect Dis 2004;39:725.
[5] Resino S, Bellon JM, Resino R, et al. Extensive implementation of highly active antiretroviral therapy shows great effect on survival and surrogate markers in vertically HIV-infected children. Clin Infect Dis 2004;38:1605.
[6] Leonard EG, McComsey GA. Metabolic complications of antiretroviral therapy in children. Pediatr Infect Dis J 2003;22:77.
[7] McComsey GA, Leonard E. Metabolic complications of HIV therapy in children. AIDS 2004;18:1753.
[8] Kingsley L, Smit E, Riddler S. Prevalence of lipodystrophy and metabolic abnormalities in the Multicenter AIDS Cohort Study (MACS). Presented at 8th Conference on Retroviruses and Opportunistic Infections. Chicago, 2001.
[9] Gripshover B, Tien PC, Saag M, et al. Lipoatrophy is the dominant feature of the lipodystrophy syndrome in HIV-infected men. Presented at 10th Conference on Retroviruses and Opportunistic Infections. Boston, 2003.
[10] Amaya R, Kozinetz C, McMeans A, Schwarzwald H, Kline M. Lipodystrophy syndrome in human immunodeficiency virus-infected children. Pediatr Infect Dis J 2002;21:405.
[11] Bitnun A, Sochett E, Babyn P, et al. Serum lipids, glucose homeostasis and abdominal adipose tissue distribution in protease inhibitor-treated and naive HIV-infected children. AIDS 2003;17:1319.
[12] Bockhorst JL, Ksseiry I, Toye M, et al. Evidence of human immunodeficiency virus-associated lipodystrophy syndrome in children treated with protease inhibitors. Pediatr Infect Dis J 2003;22:463.
[13] Brambilla P, Bricalli D, Sala N, et al. Highly active antiretroviral-treated HIV-infected children show fat distribution changes even in absence of lipodystrophy. AIDS 2001;15:2415.
[14] Jaquet D, Levine M, Ortega-Rodriguez E, et al. Clinical and metabolic presentation of the lipodystrophic syndrome in HIV-infected children. AIDS 2000;14:2123.
[15] Vigano A, Mora S, Testolin C, et al. Increased lipodystrophy is associated with increased exposure to highly active antiretroviral therapy in HIV-infected children. J Acquir Immune Defic Syndr 2003;32:482.
[16] Wedekind CA, Pugatch D. Lipodystrophy syndrome in children infected with human immunodeficiency virus. Pharmacotherapy 2001;21:861.
[17] Carr A, Samaras K, Burton S, et al. A syndrome of peripheral lipodystrophy, hyperlipidaemia and insulin resistance in patients receiving HIV protease inhibitors. AIDS 1998;12:F51.
[18] Saint-Marc T, Partisani M, Poizot-Martin I, et al. A syndrome of peripheral fat wasting (lipodystrophy) in patients receiving long-term nucleoside analogue therapy. AIDS 1999;13:1659.
[19] Galli M, Ridolfo AL, Adorni F, et al. Body habitus changes and metabolic alterations in protease inhibitor-naive HIV-1-infected patients treated with two nucleoside reverse transcriptase inhibitors. J Acquir Immune Defic Syndr 2002;29:21.
[20] Mallal SA, John M, Moore CB, James IR, McKinnon EJ. Contribution of nucleoside analogue reverse transcriptase inhibitors to subcutaneous fat wasting in patients with HIV infection. AIDS 2000;14:1309.
[21] Cohen C, Shen Y, Rode R, et al. Effect of nucleoside intensification on prevalence of morphologic abnormalities at year 5 of ritonavir plus saquinavir therapy in an HIV-infected cohort. Presented at 9th Conference on Retroviruses and Opportunistic Infections. Seattle, 2002.
[22] van der Valk M, Gisolf EH, Reiss P, et al. Increased risk of lipodystrophy when nucleoside analogue reverse transcriptase inhibitors are included with protease inhibitors in the treatment of HIV-1 infection. AIDS 2001;15:847.

[23] Galli M, Ridolfo AL, Adorni F, et al. Correlates of risk of adipose tissue alterations and their modifications over time in HIV-1-infected women treated with antiretroviral therapy. Antivir Ther 2003;8:347.

[24] Joly V, Flandre P, Meiffredy V, et al. Increased risk of lipoatrophy under stavudine in HIV-1-infected patients: results of a substudy from a comparative trial. AIDS 2002;16:2447.

[25] Podzamczer D, Ferrer E, Sanchez P, et al. Toxicity and efficacy of 3TC/EFV associated with stavudine or abacavir in antiretroviral-naive patients: 48 week results of a randomized open and multicenter trial (ABCDE) study. Presented at 11th Conference on Retroviruses and Opportunistic Infections, San Francisco.

[26] Chene G, Angelini E, Cotte L, et al. Role of long-term nucleoside-analogue therapy in lipodystrophy and metabolic disorders in human immunodeficiency virus-infected patients. Clin Infect Dis 2002;34:649.

[27] Amin J, Moore A, Carr A, et al. Combined analysis of two-year follow-up from two open-label randomized trials comparing efficacy of three nucleoside reverse transcriptase inhibitor backbones for previously untreated HIV-1 infection: OzCombo 1 and 2. HIV Clin Trials 2003;4:252.

[28] McComsey G, Bhumbra N, Ma JF, Rathore M, Alvarez A. Impact of protease inhibitor substitution with efavirenz in HIV-infected children: results of the First Pediatric Switch Study. Pediatrics 2003;111:e275.

[29] Martinez E, Garcia-Viejo MA, Blanco JL, et al. Impact of switching from human immunodeficiency virus type 1 protease inhibitors to efavirenz in successfully treated adults with lipodystrophy. Clin Infect Dis 2000;31:1266.

[30] Moyle GJ, Baldwin C, Langroudi B, Mandalia S, Gazzard BG. A 48-week, randomized, open-label comparison of three abacavir-based substitution approaches in the management of dyslipidemia and peripheral lipoatrophy. J Acquir Immune Defic Syndr 2003;33:22.

[31] Ruiz L, Negredo E, Domingo P, et al. Antiretroviral treatment simplification with nevirapine in protease inhibitor-experienced patients with HIV-associated lipodystrophy: 1-year prospective follow-up of a multicenter, randomized, controlled study. J Acquir Immune Defic Syndr 2001;27:229.

[32] Boyd M, Bien D, Van Warmerdam P, et al. Lipodystrophy in patients switched to indinavir/ritonavir 800/100 mg BID and efavirenz 600 mg QD after failing nucleoside combination therapy: a prospective, 48-week observational sub-study of HIV-NAT. Presented at 10th Conference on Retrovirused and Opportunistic Infections. Boston, 2003.

[33] McComsey GA, Ward DJ, Hessenthaler SM, et al. Improvement in lipoatrophy associated with highly active antiretroviral therapy in human immunodeficiency virus-infected patients switched from stavudine to abacavir or zidovudine: the results of the TARHEEL study. Clin Infect Dis 2004;38:263.

[34] Carr A, Workman C, Smith D, et al. Abacavir substitution for nucleoside analogs in patients with HIV lipoatrophy: a randomized trial. JAMA 2002;288:207.

[35] Despres JP, Lamarche B, Mauriege P, et al. Hyperinsulinemia as an independent risk factor for ischemic heart disease. N Engl J Med 1996;334:952.

[36] Manson JE, Colditz GA, Stampfer MJ, et al. A prospective study of obesity and risk of coronary heart disease in women. N Engl J Med 1990;322:882.

[37] Larsson B, Svardsudd K, Welin L, Wilhelmsen L, Bjorntorp P, Tibblin G. Abdominal adipose tissue distribution, obesity, and risk of cardiovascular disease and death: 13 year follow up of participants in the study of men born in 1913. BMJ (Clin Res Educ) 1984;288:1401.

[38] Howard G, Bergman R, Wagenknecht LE, et al. Ability of alternative indices of insulin sensitivity to predict cardiovascular risk: comparison with the "minimal model." Insulin Resistance Atherosclerosis Study (IRAS) investigators. Ann Epidemiol 1998;8:358.

[39] Haffner SM, Kennedy E, Gonzalez C, Stern MP, Miettinen H. A prospective analysis of the HOMA model. The Mexico City Diabetes Study. Diabetes Care 1996;19:1138.

[40] Meigs JB, D'Agostino RB Sr, Wilson PW, Cupples LA, Nathan DM, Singer DE. Risk variable clustering in the insulin resistance syndrome. The Framingham Offspring Study. Diabetes 1997;46:1594.
[41] Walton C, Lees B, Crook D, Worthington M, Godsland IF, Stevenson JC. Body fat distribution, rather than overall adiposity, influences serum lipids and lipoproteins in healthy men independently of age. Am J Med 1995;99:459.
[42] Hadigan C, Meigs JB, Wilson PW, et al. Prediction of coronary heart disease risk in HIV-infected patients with fat redistribution. Clin Infect Dis 2003;36:909.
[43] Brambilla P, Manzoni P, Sironi S, et al. Peripheral and abdominal adiposity in childhood obesity. Int J Obes Relat Metab Disord 1994;18:795.
[44] Berenson GS, Srinivasan SR, Bao W, Newman WP 3rd, Tracy RE, Wattigney WA. Association between multiple cardiovascular risk factors and atherosclerosis in children and young adults. The Bogalusa Heart Study. N Engl J Med 1998;338:1650.
[45] Goran MI, Gower BA. Relation between visceral fat and disease risk in children and adolescents. Am J Clin Nutr 1999;70:149S.
[46] Steinberger J, Daniels SR. Obesity, insulin resistance, diabetes, and cardiovascular risk in children: an American Heart Association scientific statement from the Atherosclerosis, Hypertension, and Obesity in the Young Committee (Council on Cardiovascular Disease in the Young) and the Diabetes Committee (Council on Nutrition, Physical Activity, and Metabolism). Circulation 2003;107:1448.
[47] Bozzette SA, Ake CF, Tam HK, Chang SW, Louis TA. Cardiovascular and cerebrovascular events in patients treated for human immunodeficiency virus infection. N Engl J Med 2003;348:702.
[48] Friis-Moller N, Sabin CA, Weber R, et al. Combination antiretroviral therapy and the risk of myocardial infarction. N Engl J Med 2003;349:1993.
[49] Friis-Moller N, Weber R, Reiss P, et al. Cardiovascular disease risk factors in HIV patients–association with antiretroviral therapy. Results from the DAD study. AIDS 2003; 17:1179.
[50] Mary-Krause M, Cotte L, Simon A, Partisani M, Costagliola D. Increased risk of myocardial infarction with duration of protease inhibitor therapy in HIV-infected men. AIDS 2003;17:2479.
[51] Duran S, Saves M, Spire B, et al. Failure to maintain long-term adherence to highly active antiretroviral therapy: the role of lipodystrophy. AIDS 2001;15:2441.
[52] Dukers NH, Stolte IG, Albrecht N, Coutinho RA, de Wit JB. The impact of experiencing lipodystrophy on the sexual behaviour and well-being among HIV-infected homosexual men. AIDS 2001;15:812.
[53] McComsey GA, Morrow JD. Lipid oxidative markers are significantly increased in lipoatrophy, but not in sustained asymptomatic hyperlactatemia. J Acquir Immune Defic Syndr 2003;34:45.
[54] McComsey G, Southwell H, Gripshover B, Salata R, Valdez H. Effects of antioxidants on plasma lipids and peripheral fat in HIV-infected subjects with lipoatrophy. J Acquir Immune Defic Syndr 2003;33:605.
[55] Gelato MC, Mynarcik DC, Quick JL, et al. Improved insulin sensitivity and body fat distribution in HIV-infected patients treated with rosiglitazone: a pilot study. J Acquir Immune Defic Syndr 2002;31:163.
[56] Hadigan C, Yawetz S, Thomas A, Havers F, Sax PE, Grinspoon S. Metabolic effects of rosiglitazone in HIV lipodystrophy: a randomized, controlled trial. Ann Intern Med 2004; 140:786.
[57] Carr A, Workman C, Carey D, et al. No effect of rosiglitazone for treatment of HIV-1 lipoatrophy: randomised, double-blind, placebo-controlled trial. Lancet 2004;363:429.
[58] Sutinen J, Hakkinen AM, Westerbacka J, et al. Rosiglitazone in the treatment of HAART associated lipodystrophy: a randomized double-blind, placebo-controlled study. Antivir Ther 2003;8:199.

[59] Rietschel P, Hadigan C, Corcoran C, et al. Assessment of growth hormone dynamics in human immunodeficiency virus-related lipodystrophy. J Clin Endocrinol Metab 2001;86: 504.

[60] Vigano A, Mora S, Brambilla P, et al. Impaired growth hormone secretion correlates with visceral adiposity in highly active antiretroviral treated HIV-infected adolescents. AIDS 2003;17:1435.

[61] Kotler DP, Grunfeld C, Muurahainen N, et al. Low-dose maintenance therapy with recombinant human growth hormone sustains effects of previous r-hGH treatment in HIV + patients with excess center fat: treatment results at 60 weeks. Presented at 11th Conference on Retroviruses and Opportunistic Infections. San Francisco.

[62] Engelson ES, Glesby MJ, Mendez D, et al. Effect of recombinant human growth hormone in the treatment of visceral fat accumulation in HIV infection. J Acquir Immune Defic Syndr 2002;30:379.

[63] Grunfeld C, Kotler DP, Hamadeh R, Tierney A, Wang J, Pierson RN. Hypertriglyceridemia in the acquired immunodeficiency syndrome. Am J Med 1989;86:27.

[64] Thiebaut R, Daucourt V, Mercie P, et al. Lipodystrophy, metabolic disorders, and human immunodeficiency virus infection: Aquitaine Cohort, France, 1999. Groupe d'Epidemiologie Clinique du Syndrome d'Immunodeficience Acquise en Aquitaine. Clin Infect Dis 2000;31:1482.

[65] Carr A, Samaras K, Thorisdottir A, Kaufmann GR, Chisholm DJ, Cooper DA. Diagnosis, prediction, and natural course of HIV-1 protease-inhibitor-associated lipodystrophy, hyperlipidaemia, and diabetes mellitus: a cohort study. Lancet 1999; 353:2093.

[66] Tsiodras S, Mantzoros C, Hammer S, Samore M. Effects of protease inhibitors on hyperglycemia, hyperlipidemia, and lipodystrophy: a 5-year cohort study. Arch Intern Med 2000;160:2050.

[67] Wanke CA. Epidemiological and clinical aspects of the metabolic complications of HIV infection the fat redistribution syndrome. AIDS 1999;13:1287.

[68] Mulligan K, Grunfeld C, Tai VW, et al. Hyperlipidemia and insulin resistance are induced by protease inhibitors independent of changes in body composition in patients with HIV infection. J Acquir Immune Defic Syndr 2000;23:35.

[69] Noor MA, Lo JC, Mulligan K, et al. Metabolic effects of indinavir in healthy HIV-seronegative men. AIDS 2001;15:F11.

[70] Purnell JQ, Zambon A, Knopp RH, et al. Effect of ritonavir on lipids and post-heparin lipase activities in normal subjects. AIDS 2000;14:51.

[71] Arpadi SM, Cuff PA, Horlick M, Wang J, Kotler DP. Lipodystrophy in HIV-infected children is associated with high viral load and low CD4+ -lymphocyte count and CD4+ -lymphocyte percentage at baseline and use of protease inhibitors and stavudine. J Acquir Immune Defic Syndr 2001;27:30.

[72] Farley J, Gona P, Crain M, Cervia J, Lindsey J, Oleske J. Prevalence of hypercholesterolemia and associated risk factors among perinatally HIV-infected children (4–19 years) in PACTG 219C. Presented at 10th Conference on Retroviruses and Opportunistic Infections. Boston, 2003.

[73] Ramos J, Garcia L, Rojo P, et al. High prevalence of metabolic abnormalities in HIV infected children treated with HAART. Presented at 10th Conference on Retroviruses and Opportunistic Infections. Boston, 2003.

[74] Gunter E, Lewis B, Koncikowski S. Laboratory procedures used for the third National Health and Nutrition Examination Survey (NHANES III), 1988–1994. Hyatsville (MD): US Department of Health and Human Services. National Center for Health Statistics. 1996. p. VIIQ1–VIIQ20.

[75] Mueller BU, Nelson RP Jr, Sleasman J, et al. A phase I/II study of the protease inhibitor ritonavir in children with human immunodeficiency virus infection. Pediatrics 1998;101: 335.

[76] Funk MB, Linde R, Wintergerst U, et al. Preliminary experiences with triple therapy including nelfinavir and two reverse transcriptase inhibitors in previously untreated HIV-infected children. AIDS 1999;13:1653.
[77] Cheseaux JJ, Jotterand V, Aebi C, et al. Hyperlipidemia in HIV-infected children treated with protease inhibitors: relevance for cardiovascular diseases. J Acquir Immune Defic Syndr 2002;30:288.
[78] Dube MP, Stein JH, Aberg JA, et al. Guidelines for the evaluation and management of dyslipidemia in human immunodeficiency virus (HIV)-infected adults receiving antiretroviral therapy: recommendations of the HIV Medical Association of the Infectious Disease Society of America and the Adult AIDS Clinical Trials Group. Clin Infect Dis 2003;37:613.
[79] Executive Summary of the Third Report of the National Cholesterol Education Program (NCEP) Expert Panel on Detection, Evaluation, and Treatment of High Blood Cholesterol in Adults (Adult Treatment Panel III). JAMA 2001;285:2486.
[80] Wierzbicki AS, Reynolds TM, Crook MA, Tatler J, Peters BS. Lipid lowering therapy in patients with HIV infection. Lancet 1998;352:1782.
[81] Penzak SR, Chuck SK. Management of protease inhibitor-associated hyperlipidemia. Am J Cardiovasc Drugs 2002;2:91.
[82] Stein EA, Illingworth DR, Kwiterovich PO Jr, et al. Efficacy and safety of lovastatin in adolescent males with heterozygous familial hypercholesterolemia: a randomized controlled trial. JAMA 1999;281:137.
[83] American Academy of Pediatrics Committee on Nutrition. Cholesterol in childhood. Pediatrics 1998;101:141.
[84] Martinez E, Conget I, Lozano L, Casamitjana R, Gatell JM. Reversion of metabolic abnormalities after switching from HIV-1 protease inhibitors to nevirapine. AIDS 1999;13:805.
[85] Negredo E, Ribalta J, Paredes R, et al. Reversal of atherogenic lipoprotein profile in HIV-1 infected patients with lipodystrophy after replacing protease inhibitors by nevirapine. AIDS 2002;16:1383.
[86] Protease inhibitors may increase blood glucose in hiv patients. Washington (DC): US Food and Drug Administration; 1997.
[87] Anderson RL, Hamman RF, Savage PJ, et al. Exploration of simple insulin sensitivity measures derived from frequently sampled intravenous glucose tolerance (FSIGT) tests. The Insulin Resistance Atherosclerosis Study. Am J Epidemiol 1995;142:724.
[88] Walli R, Herfort O, Michl GM, et al. Treatment with protease inhibitors associated with peripheral insulin resistance and impaired oral glucose tolerance in HIV-1-infected patients. AIDS 1998;12:F167.
[89] Behrens G, Dejam A, Schmidt H, et al. Impaired glucose tolerance, beta cell function and lipid metabolism in HIV patients under treatment with protease inhibitors. AIDS 1999;13:F63.
[90] Murata H, Hruz PW, Mueckler M. Indinavir inhibits the glucose transporter isoform Glut4 at physiologic concentrations. AIDS 2002;16:859.
[91] Rudich A, Vanounou S, Riesenberg K, et al. The HIV protease inhibitor nelfinavir induces insulin resistance and increases basal lipolysis in 3T3–L1 adipocytes. Diabetes 2001;50:1425.
[92] Hadigan C, Borgonha S, Rabe J, Young V, Grinspoon S. Increased rates of lipolysis among human immunodeficiency virus-infected men receiving highly active antiretroviral therapy. Metabolism 2002;51:1143.
[93] Hadigan C, Meigs JB, Corcoran C, et al. Metabolic abnormalities and cardiovascular disease risk factors in adults with human immunodeficiency virus infection and lipodystrophy. Clin Infect Dis 2001;32:130.
[94] Kosmiski LA, Kuritzkes DR, Lichtenstein KA, et al. Fat distribution and metabolic changes are strongly correlated and energy expenditure is increased in the HIV lipodystrophy syndrome. AIDS 2001;15:1993.

[95] Meininger G, Hadigan C, Rietschel P, Grinspoon S. Body-composition measurements as predictors of glucose and insulin abnormalities in HIV-positive men. Am J Clin Nutr 2002; 76:460.
[96] Cook JS, Hoffman RP, Stene MA, Hansen JR. Effects of maturational stage on insulin sensitivity during puberty. J Clin Endocrinol Metab 1993;77:725.
[97] Travers SH, Jeffers BW, Bloch CA, Hill JO, Eckel RH. Gender and Tanner stage differences in body composition and insulin sensitivity in early pubertal children. J Clin Endocrinol Metab 1995;80:172.
[98] Hadigan C, Jeste S, Anderson EJ, Tsay R, Cyr H, Grinspoon S. Modifiable dietary habits and their relation to metabolic abnormalities in men and women with human immunodeficiency virus infection and fat redistribution. Clin Infect Dis 2001;33:710.
[99] Thoni GJ, Fedou C, Brun JF, et al. Reduction of fat accumulation and lipid disorders by individualized light aerobic training in human immunodeficiency virus infected patients with lipodystrophy and/or dyslipidemia. Diabetes Metab 2002;28:397.
[100] Hadigan C, Rabe J, Grinspoon S. Sustained benefits of metformin therapy on markers of cardiovascular risk in human immunodeficiency virus-infected patients with fat redistribution and insulin resistance. J Clin Endocrinol Metab 2002;87:4611.
[101] Hadigan C, Corcoran C, Basgoz N, Davis B, Sax P, Grinspoon S. Metformin in the treatment of HIV lipodystrophy syndrome: a randomized controlled trial. JAMA 2000; 284:472.
[102] Saint-Marc T, Touraine JL. Effects of metformin on insulin resistance and central adiposity in patients receiving effective protease inhibitor therapy. AIDS 1999;13:1000.
[103] Inzucchi SE, Maggs DG, Spollett GR, et al. Efficacy and metabolic effects of metformin and troglitazone in type II diabetes mellitus. N Engl J Med 1998;338:867.
[104] Maggs DG, Buchanan TA, Burant CF, et al. Metabolic effects of troglitazone monotherapy in type 2 diabetes mellitus: a randomized, double-blind, placebo-controlled trial. Ann Intern Med 1998;128:176.
[105] Miller KD, Masur H, Jones EC, et al. High prevalence of osteonecrosis of the femoral head in HIV-infected adults. Ann Intern Med 2002;137:17.
[106] Gaughan DM, Mofenson LM, Hughes MD, Seage GR 3rd, Ciupak GL, Oleske JM. Osteonecrosis of the hip (Legg-Calve-Perthes disease) in human immunodeficiency virus-infected children. Pediatrics 2002;109:E74.
[107] Keruly JC, Chaisson RE, Moore RD. Increasing incidence of avascular necrosis of the hip in HIV-infected patients. J Acquir Immune Defic Syndr 2001;28:101.
[108] Glesby MJ, Hoover DR, Vaamonde CM. Osteonecrosis in patients infected with human immunodeficiency virus: a case-control study. J Infect Dis 2001;184:519.
[109] Brown P, Crane L. Avascular necrosis of bone in patients with human immunodeficiency virus infection: report of 6 cases and review of the literature. Clin Infect Dis 2001;32:1221.
[110] Lawal A, Engelson ES, Wang J, Heymsfield SB, Kotler DP. Equivalent osteopenia in HIV-infected individuals studied before and during the era of highly active antiretroviral therapy. AIDS 2001;15:278.
[111] Mondy K, Yarasheski K, Powderly WG, et al. Longitudinal evolution of bone mineral density and bone markers in human immunodeficiency virus-infected individuals. Clin Infect Dis 2003;36:482.
[112] Bruera D, Luna N, David DO, Bergoglio LM, Zamudio J. Decreased bone mineral density in HIV-infected patients is independent of antiretroviral therapy. AIDS 2003;17:1917.
[113] McGowan J, Cheng A, Coleman S, Johnson A, Genant H. Assessment of bone mineral density (BMD) in HIV-infected antiretroviral therapy naive subjects. Presented at 8th Conference on Retroviruses and Opportunistic Infections. Chicago, 2001.
[114] Ramos J, Rojo P, Ruano C, et al. Stability of osteopenia in HIV-infected children over time. Presented at 11th Conference on Retrovirus and Opportunistic Infections. San Francisco.

[115] McComsey G, Leonard E. The effect of calcium and vitamin D on bone mineral density in HIV-infected children with osteoporosis. Presented at 10th Conference on Retroviruses and Opportunistic Infections. Boston, 2003.
[116] Mosekilde L. Sex differences in age-related loss of vertebral trabecular bone mass and structure–biomechanical consequences. Bone 1989;10:425.
[117] Lawal A, Engelson E, Wang J, Heymsefield S, Kotler D. Effect of oxandrolone upon bone mineral content in malnourished HIV + patients. Presented at 8th Conference on Retroviruses and Opportunistic Infections. Chicago, 2001.
[118] Lawal A, Engelson E, Wang J, Heymsfield SB, Kotler D. Effect of growth hormone on osteopenia in HIV + patients. Presented at 8th Conference on Retroviruses and Opportunistic Infections. Chicago, 2001.
[119] Mondy K, Powderly WG, Claxton S, et al. Alendronate, vitamin D, and calcium for the treatment of osteopenia/osteoporosis associated with HIV infection. Presented at 10th Conference on Retroviruses and Opportunistic Infections. Boston, 2003.
[120] Guaraldi G, Orlando G, Madeddu G, et al. Alendronate reduces bone turnover in HIV-associated osteopenia and osteoporosis. Presented at 11th Conference on Retrovirus and Opportunistic Infections. San Francisco.
[121] Chattha G, Arieff AI, Cummings C, Tierney LM Jr. Lactic acidosis complicating the acquired immunodeficiency syndrome. Ann Intern Med 1993;118:37.
[122] Freiman JP, Helfert KE, Hamrell MR, Stein DS. Hepatomegaly with severe steatosis in HIV-seropositive patients. AIDS 1993;7:379.
[123] Gerard Y, Maulin L, Yazdanpanah Y, et al. Symptomatic hyperlactataemia: an emerging complication of antiretroviral therapy. AIDS 2000;14:2723.
[124] Chariot P, Drogou I, de Lacroix-Szmania I, et al. Zidovudine-induced mitochondrial disorder with massive liver steatosis, myopathy, lactic acidosis, and mitochondrial DNA depletion. J Hepatol 1999;30:156.
[125] Fortgang IS, Belitsos PC, Chaisson RE, Moore RD. Hepatomegaly and steatosis in HIV-infected patients receiving nucleoside analog antiretroviral therapy. Am J Gastroenterol 1995;90:1433.
[126] ter Hofstede HJ, de Marie S, Foudraine NA, Danner SA, Brinkman K. Clinical features and risk factors of lactic acidosis following long-term antiretroviral therapy: 4 fatal cases. Int J Sex Transm Dis AIDS 2000;11:611.
[127] Lonergan JT, Havlir D, Barber E, Matthews WC. Incidence and outcome of hyper-lactatemia associated with clinical manifestations in HIV-infected adults receiving NRTI-containing regimens. Presented at 8th Conference on Retroviruses and Opportunistic Infections. Chicago, 2001.
[128] Blanche S, Tardieu M, Rustin P, et al. Persistent mitochondrial dysfunction and perinatal exposure to antiretroviral nucleoside analogues. Lancet 1999;354:1084.
[129] Barret B, Tardieu M, Rustin P, et al. Persistent mitochondrial dysfunction in HIV-1-exposed but uninfected infants: clinical screening in a large prospective cohort. AIDS 2003; 17:1769.
[130] Gianquinto C, Rampon O, Torresan S, et al. Lactic acid levels in infants exposed to ART during fetal life. Presented at 11th Conference on Retroviruses and Opportunistic Infections. San Francisco.
[131] Alimenti A, Ogilvie G, Burdge D, Money D, Forbes J. Lactic acidemia in infants exposed to perinatal antiretroviral therapy. Presented at 9th Conference on Retroviruses and Opportunistic Infections. Seattle, 2002.
[132] Brinkman K, Troost N, Schrijnders L, et al. Usefulness of routine lactate measurement to prevent lactic acidosis: evaluation of a protocol. Presented at 9th Conference on Retroviruses and Opportunistic Infections. Seattle, 2002.
[133] McComsey G, Yau L. Asymptomatic hyperlactatemia: predictive value, natural history and correlates. Antivir Ther 2004;9:205.

[134] Desai N, Mathur M, Weedon J. Lactate levels in children with HIV/AIDS on highly active antiretroviral therapy. AIDS 2003;17:1565.
[135] Noguera A, Fortuny C, Sanchez E, et al. Hyperlactatemia in human immunodeficiency virus-infected children receiving antiretroviral treatment. Pediatr Infect Dis J 2003;22:778.
[136] Lonergan JT, Barber RE, Mathews WC. Safety and efficacy of switching to alternative nucleoside analogues following symptomatic hyperlactatemia and lactic acidosis. AIDS 2003;17:2495.
[137] Lonergan JT, McComsey G, Fisher R, et al. Lack of recurrence of hyperlactatemia in HIV-infected patients switched from stavudine to abacavir or zidovudine. J Acquir Immune Defic Syndr 2004;36:935.
[138] Ribera E, Sauleda S, Paradineiro J, et al. Increase in mitochondrial DNA in PBMCs and improvement of lipid profile and lactate levels in patients with lipoatrophy when stavudine is switched to tenofovir. Presented at 9th European AIDS Conference. Warsaw, Poland, 2003.

ELSEVIER
SAUNDERS

INFECTIOUS
DISEASE CLINICS
OF NORTH AMERICA

Infect Dis Clin N Am 19 (2005) 731–745

The Treatment of Children Exposed to Pathogens Linked to Bioterrorism

David Markenson, MD, EMT-P[a,b,*]

[a]Division of Pediatric Critical Care, Department of Pediatrics, Flushing Hospital Medical Center, 4500 Parsons Boulevard, Flushing, NY 11355, USA
[b]National Center for Disaster Preparedness, Columbia University Mailman School of Public Health, 722 West 168th Street, 10th Floor, New York, NY 10032, USA

Bioterrorism preparedness is a highly specific component of general emergency preparedness. In addition to the unique pediatric issues involved in general emergency preparedness, terrorism preparedness must consider several additional issues, including the unique vulnerabilities of children to various agents and the limited availability of age-appropriate and weight-appropriate antidotes and treatments. Although children may respond more rapidly to therapeutic intervention, they also are more susceptible to various agents and conditions and more likely to deteriorate if not monitored carefully.

The release of chemical or biologic toxins would affect children disproportionately through several mechanisms. Because children become dehydrated easily and possess minimal reserve, they are at greater risk than adults when exposed to agents that may cause diarrhea or vomiting. Agents that might cause only mild symptoms in an adult could lead to hypovolemic shock in an infant. Another example involves the unique respiratory physiology of children. Many of the agents used for chemical and biologic attacks are aerosolized (eg, sarin, chlorine, or anthrax). Because children have faster respiratory rates than adults, they are exposed to relatively greater dosages and experience the effects of these agents much more rapidly than adults. Many biologic and chemical agents are absorbed through the skin. Because children have more permeable skin and more surface area relative to body mass than adults, they receive proportionally higher doses of agents that either affect the skin or are absorbed through the skin. In

* Columbia University Mailman School of Public Health, 722 West 168th Street, 10th Floor, New York, NY 10032, USA.
E-mail address: dsm2002@columbia.edu

0891-5520/05/$ - see front matter
doi:10.1016/j.idc.2005.05.004 *id.theclinics.com*

addition, because the skin of children is poorly keratinized, vesicants and corrosives result in greater injury to children than to adults.

It is well known that children may exhibit different effects of biologic agents, as follows:

- Smallpox—children lack immunity, whereas some adults who were vaccinated as children still may possess some degree of immunity
- Trichothecenes—children may be more susceptible
- Melioidosis—children manifest unique parotitis
- Anthrax—children are less susceptible to the effects of anthrax

In addition to the differences in clinical presentation of biologic agents, children may present different incubation periods after exposure. For many agents, the incubation period is shorter for children. Consequently, surveillance systems based on symptoms in children may yield earlier detection, which can lead to earlier containment and mitigate the effects of a bioterrorism agent.

Lastly, there may be issues with the antibiotics of choice for bioterrorist agents. Many medications that are used in children are not approved by the US Food and Drug Administration (FDA) for such use. Although this situation does not pose a problem for health care providers, several government programs, such as the Strategic National Stockpile, may stock items only for the FDA-approved indications. In addition, certain medications may have an absolute contraindication to use in children, whereas others may have relative contraindications.

Biologic weapons are referred to as the "poor man's nuclear bomb" because they are easy to manufacture, can be deployed without sophisticated delivery systems, and have the ability to kill or injure hundreds of thousands of people. Various biologic agents could be used as weapons, and the actual clinical syndrome varies depending on the type of agent, its virulence, route of exposure, and susceptibility of the victim to infection. In contrast to chemical, conventional, and nuclear weapons that generate immediate effects, biologic agents generally are associated with a delay in the onset of illness and may not be recognized in their initial stages. A covert release of a contagious biologic agent has the potential for large-scale spread before detection (which depends on traditional disease surveillance methods). For some infectious agents, secondary and tertiary transmission may continue for weeks or months after the initial attack. In an epidemic, overwhelming numbers of critically ill patients require acute and follow-up medical care. Infected persons and the "worried well" seek medical attention, with a corresponding need for medical supplies, diagnostic tests, and hospital beds. Simple devices, such as crop dusting airplanes or small perfume atomizers, are effective delivery systems for biologic agents.

Biologic weapon releases on civilian populations also have occurred in the recent past. In 1984 in Oregon, approximately 750 people experienced salmonellosis after bacteria were spread on salad bars in an effort to disrupt local elections. An inadvertent release of anthrax in April 1979 by a military facility in Sverdlovsk, in the former USSR, produced mass infection 50 km away, with 66 documented deaths.

As a weapon, biologic agents possess a marked diversity in the type of injury produced by infectious agents, with toxic effects ranging from incapacitation to death. The biologic agents listed in Box 1 are considered to be likely candidates for weaponization. Box 1 includes agents that may be classified as bacteria, viruses, rickettsia, fungi, and preformed toxins.

The Centers for Disease Control and Prevention separates bioterrorist agents into three categories (A, B, and C) in order of priority based on the combined factors of availability, potential for morbidity and mortality, and ease of dissemination (Table 1). Although virtually any microorganism has the potential to be used as a biologic weapon, most would be difficult to weaponize and disseminate effectively. Although the microorganisms listed in Box 1 are possible candidates for weaponization, the biologic agents most likely to be used as possible terrorist agents are *Bacillus anthracis* (anthrax), *Brucella* species (brucellosis), *Clostridium botulinum* (botulism), *Francisella tularensis* (tularemia), *Yersinia pestis* (plague), Ebola virus, variola (smallpox), the hemorrhagic fever viruses, and *Coxiella burnetii* (Q fever).

Bacterial agents

Anthrax

Anthrax has been extensively developed as a biologic weapon and is considered the most likely candidate for a biologic release. More recent history in New York City, Connecticut, and Florida has shown that the use of anthrax as a terrorism agent is not a theoretical possibility, but a reality. The causative organism, *B anthracis,* is a gram-positive sporulating rod. Anthrax cannot be transmitted through person-to-person contact. Because the initial symptoms of anthrax are nonspecific, and physician experience with the disease is uncommon, anthrax may be misdiagnosed.

Most experts believe that a bioterrorist attack using anthrax most likely would involve aerosol exposure. The incubation period for inhalation anthrax is usually less than 1 week, but there have been cases with incubation periods of 30 days. The first indication of an aerosol exposure may be groups of patients presenting with severe influenza-like disease with a high case-fatality rate. After a few hours or days, and possibly some improvement, the condition progresses to fever, dyspnea, and eventually shock. A widened mediastinum consistent with lymphadenopathy or hemorrhagic mediastinitis is common. Usually, no evidence of bronchopneumonia exists. The symptoms (warning signs) of anthrax are different depending on the type of the disease (Box 2).

Box 1. Biologic agents considered to be likely candidates for weaponization

Bacteria

Bacillus anthracis (anthrax)
Brucella abortus, B melitensis, B suis (brucellosis)
Burkholderia mallei, B pseudomallei
Clostridium botulinum (botulism)
Francisella tularensis (tularemia)
Yersinia pestis (plague)

Viruses

Crimean-Congo hemorrhagic fever
Eastern equine encephalitis virus
Ebola virus
Equine morbillivirus
Lassa fever virus
Marburg virus
Rift Valley fever virus
South American hemorrhagic fever virus
Tick-borne encephalitis complex
Variola (smallpox)
Venezuelan equine encephalitis virus
Hantavirus
Yellow fever virus

Rickettsia

Coxiella burnetii (Q fever)
Rickettsia prowazekii (epidemic typhus)
Rickettsia rickettsii (Rocky Mountain spotted fever)

Fungi

Coccidioides immitis (coccidioidomycosis)

Toxins

Abrun
Aflatoxin
Botulinum toxins
Clostridium perfringens epsilon toxin
Conotoxin
Diacetoxyscirpenol
Ricin

Table 1
Centers for Disease Control and Prevention categories, definitions, and pathogens

Category	CDC definition	Pathogens
A	High-priority agents include organisms that pose a risk to national security because they: Can be disseminated or transmitted easily from person to person Result in high mortality rates and have the potential for major public health impact Might cause public panic and social disruption Require special action for public health preparedness	Anthrax (*Bacillus anthracis*) Botulism (*Clostridium botulinum* toxin) Plague (*Yersinia pestis*) Smallpox (variola major) Tularemia (*Francisella tularensis*) Viral hemorrhagic fevers (filoviruses [eg, Ebola, Marburg] and arenaviruses [eg, Lassa, Machupo])
B	Second highest priority agents include those that Are moderately easy to disseminate Result in moderate morbidity rates and low mortality rates Require specific enhancements of CDC's diagnostic capacity and enhanced disease surveillance	Brucellosis (*Brucella*) Epsilon toxin of *Clostridium perfringens* Food safety threats (eg, *Salmonella*, *Escherichia coli* O157:H7, *Shigella*) Glanders (*Burkholderia mallei*) Melioidosis (*Burkholderia pseudomallei*) Psittacosis (*Chlamydia psittaci*) Q fever (*Coxiella burnetii*) Ricin toxin from *Ricinus communis* (castor beans) Staphylococcal enterotoxin B Typhus fever (*Rickettsia prowazekii*) Viral encephalitis (alphaviruses [eg, Venezuelan equine encephalitis, eastern equine encephalitis, western equine encephalitis]) Water safety threats (eg, *Vibrio cholerae*, *Cryptosporidium parvum*)
C	Third highest priority agents include emerging pathogens that could be engineered for mass dissemination in the future because of Availability Ease of production and dissemination Potential for high morbidity and mortality rates and major health impact	Emerging infectious diseases, such as Nipah virus and hantavirus

Adapted from Centers for Disease Control and Prevention. Biological and chemical terrorism: strategic plan for preparedness and response. MMWR 2000;49:1–14.

Although *treatment* is unlikely to be effective after the patient becomes ill, it can prevent patients from becoming sick if begun soon after exposure. Terrorists likely would use strains that are resistant to penicillin or doxycycline, so quinolones would be preferred until susceptibility is

Box 2. Symptoms of anthrax

Cutaneous
The first symptom is a small sore that develops into a blister. The blister develops into a skin ulcer with a black area in the center. The sore, blister, and ulcer do not hurt.

Gastrointestinal
The first symptoms are nausea, loss of appetite, bloody diarrhea, and fever, followed by severe stomach pain.

Inhalation
The first symptoms of inhalation anthrax are similar to cold or flu symptoms and include a sore throat, mild fever, and muscle aches. Later symptoms include cough, chest discomfort, shortness of breath, tiredness, and muscle aches.

known. As a result, treatment for confirmed inhalation cases includes a combination of agents, particularly either ciprofloxacin or doxycycline, along with clindamycin and penicillin G. Patients who are stable after 14 days can be switched to a single oral agent to complete a 60-day course of therapy.

The preferred *prophylactic* regimen includes administration of vaccine (three times at 0, 2, and 4 weeks) and antibiotics (ciprofloxin or doxycycline) for 30 days. The anthrax vaccine is currently in limited supply, and if it is not available, antibiotics should be given for 60 days because spores can persist in tissues for a long time. The choice of ciprofloxacin as the initial agent for prophylaxis is based on the belief that weaponized anthrax is most likely going to be a resistant strain. Other quinolones (eg, levofloxacin, moxifloxacin, gatifloxacin) also are assumed to be effective. Despite ciprofloxacin being the only drug approved for prophylaxis against aerosol anthrax, its use in children has been questioned because of a theoretical risk of cartilage damage from animal studies. It is still recommended that ciprofloxacin be used in children as the initial prophylactic agent, however, simply because the possibility of resistant strains is high. If the strain ultimately is found to be sensitive, amoxicillin can be used as an alternative for the remainder of the course of treatment. Based on current information, an amoxicillin dosage of at least 45 mg/kg/d, divided into three doses (ie, 15 mg/kg) and given every 8 hours to children weighing less than 40 kg, should result in adequate plasma concentrations for susceptible isolates of *B anthracis* for 75% to 100% of the dosing interval. Daily dosages of less than 45 mg/kg and dosing intervals greater than every 8 hours should not be used for prophylaxis of postexposure inhalational anthrax.

Plague

Plague, caused by *Y pestis,* also is considered a potential bacterial weapon. In contrast to anthrax, pneumonic plague can be highly contagious, and if untreated, mortality can be 100%. The pneumonic form of plague would be the primary form seen after purposeful aerosol dissemination of the organism. The bubonic form would be seen after purposeful dissemination through the release of infected fleas. The typical sign of the most common form of human plague is a swollen and very tender lymph gland, accompanied by pain. The swollen gland is called a "bubo." Bubonic plague should be suspected when a person develops a swollen gland, fever, chills, headache, and extreme exhaustion and has a history of possible exposure to infected rodents, rabbits, or fleas. A person usually becomes ill with bubonic plague 2 to 6 days after being infected. When bubonic plague is left untreated, plague bacteria invade the bloodstream. As the plague bacteria multiply in the bloodstream, they spread rapidly throughout the body and cause a severe and often fatal condition. Infection of the lungs with the plague bacterium causes the pneumonic form of plague, a severe respiratory illness. The infected person may experience high fever, chills, cough, and breathing difficulty and may expel bloody sputum. If plague patients are not given specific antibiotic therapy, the disease can progress rapidly to death. Recovery from the disease may be followed by temporary immunity. The organism probably remains viable in water and moist meals and grains for several weeks.

Tularemia

Tularemia, a bacterial zoonosis, is caused by *F tularensis,* one of the most infectious pathogenic bacteria known. It requires inoculation or inhalation of only 10 organisms to cause disease. *F tularensis* could be used as a biologic weapon in numerous ways, but an aerosol release likely would have the greatest adverse medical and public health consequences. Airborne *F tularensis* would be expected principally to cause pleuropneumonitis, but some exposures might contaminate the eye, resulting in ocular tularemia; penetrate broken skin, resulting in ulceroglandular or glandular disease; or cause oropharyngeal disease with cervical lymphadenitis. *F tularensis* can infect humans through the skin, mucous membranes, gastrointestinal tract, and lungs. Primary clinical forms vary in severity and presentation according to virulence of the infecting organism, dose, and site of inoculum. The onset of tularemia is usually abrupt, with fever (38–40°C), headache, chills and rigors, generalized body aches (often prominent in the low back), coryza, and sore throat. A dry or slightly productive cough and substernal pain or tightness frequently occur with or without objective signs of pneumonia, such as purulent sputum, dyspnea, tachypnea, pleuritic pain, or hemoptysis. Nausea, vomiting, and diarrhea may occur. Humans with inhalational exposures also develop hemorrhagic inflammation of the airways early in the course of illness, which may progress to bronchopneumonia.

Because it is unknown whether drug-resistant organisms might be used in a bioterrorist event, antimicrobial susceptibility testing of isolates should be conducted quickly and treatments altered according to test results and clinical responses. Streptomycin is the drug of choice, but is available only for compassionate usage and in limited supplies. Gentamicin, which is more widely available and can be used intravenously, is an acceptable alternative. Tetracyclines and chloramphenicol also can be used, but relapses and primary treatment failures occur at a higher rate with these bacteriostatic agents than with aminoglycosides, and they would pose a problem for pediatric patients.

Viral agents

Viruses of concern include variola (smallpox), Ebola and other hemorrhagic viruses, and the viral encephalitides.

Smallpox

There are two clinical forms of smallpox. Variola major is the severe and most common form of smallpox, with a more extensive rash and higher fever. There are four types of variola major smallpox: ordinary (the most frequent type, accounting for $\geq$90% of cases), modified (mild and occurring in previously vaccinated persons), flat, and hemorrhagic (rare and very severe). Historically, variola major has an overall fatality rate of about 30%; however, flat and hemorrhagic smallpox usually are fatal. Variola minor is a less common presentation of smallpox and a much less severe disease, with death rates historically of 1% or less. A patient with smallpox is sometimes contagious with onset of fever (prodrome phase), but the patient becomes most contagious with the onset of rash. The infected patient is contagious until the last smallpox scab falls off. Generally, direct and fairly prolonged face-to-face contact is required to spread smallpox from one patient to another. Smallpox also can be spread through direct contact with infected bodily fluids or contaminated objects, such as bedding or clothing. Rarely, smallpox has been spread by virus carried in the air in enclosed settings such as buildings, buses, and trains. Humans are the only natural hosts of variola. Smallpox is not known to be transmitted by insects or animals.

Exposure to the virus is followed by an incubation period during which patients do not have any symptoms and may feel fine. This incubation period averages about 12 to 14 days (range 7–17 days). During this time, patients are not contagious. A rash emerges first as small red spots on the tongue and in the mouth. These spots develop into sores that break open and spread large amounts of the virus into the mouth and throat. At this time, the patient becomes most contagious. Around the time the sores in the mouth break down, a rash appears on the skin, starting on the face and spreading to the arms and legs and then to the hands and feet. Usually the rash spreads to all parts of the body within 24 hours. As the rash appears, the fever usually decreases, and the patient may start to feel better. By the third day of the rash, the rash becomes raised bumps. By the fourth day, the bumps fill with a thick, opaque fluid and often have a depression in the center that looks like a bellybutton. (This is a major distinguishing characteristic of smallpox.) Fever often increases again at this time and remains high until scabs form over the bumps. The bumps become pustules—sharply raised, usually round and firm to the touch as if there is a small round object under the skin. The pustules begin to form a crust and then scab. By the end of the second week after the rash appears, most of the sores have scabbed over. Most scabs have fallen off 3 weeks after the rash appears. The patient is contagious to others until all of the scabs have fallen off.

Because smallpox was eradicated globally in 1980, and children are no longer being immunized, more than 80% of the adult population and 100% of children are susceptible to variola virus. The Centers for Disease Control and Prevention currently recommends against vaccination of children younger than 1 year. In reality, all contraindications to smallpox vaccination are relative. After bona fide exposure, vaccination of even the youngest infants should be done.

Viral hemorrhagic fevers

The viral hemorrhagic fevers are a diverse group of illnesses that are due to RNA viruses of several different viral families: the Filoviridae, including the Ebola and Marburg viruses; the Arenaviridae, including Lassa fever and the Argentinean and Bolivian hemorrhagic fever viruses; the Bunyaviridae, including various hantaviruses, Crimean-Congo hemorrhagic fever virus, and Rift Valley fever virus (a phlebovirus); and the Flaviviridae, including yellow fever virus, Dengue hemorrhagic fever virus, and others. In general, the term *viral hemorrhagic fever* is used to describe a viral infection that causes a severe multisystem syndrome characterized by overall damage to the vascular system with a compromise of the body's ability to regulate itself. These systemic effects often are accompanied by hemorrhage (bleeding); however, the bleeding itself is rarely life-threatening. Although some types of hemorrhagic fever viruses can cause relatively mild illnesses, many of these viruses cause severe, life-threatening disease. Although evidence of weaponization does not exist for many of these viruses, they should be considered in terrorism preparedness because of their *potential* for weaponization or aerosol dissemination.

Toxins

Toxins derived from biologic agents generally have the characteristics of chemical agents, producing illness within hours of exposure. Although the effects of these agents can be significant, these agents are not contagious.

Botulinum toxin

Botulinum toxin is produced by the bacterium *C botulinum*; it is one of the most potent toxins known and is 100,000 times more toxic than sarin. When inhaled, these toxins produce a clinical picture similar to that of food-borne intoxication, although the time to onset of paralytic signs may be longer and may vary by type and dose of toxin. Treatment is available in the form of a trivalent antitoxin (types A, B, and E), and there is a pentavalent immunoglobulin (types A through E) available in limited supply for treatment of infantile botulism.

Staphylococcal enterotoxin

The enterotoxin of *Staphylococcus aureus* is also incapacitating, although not highly lethal except in elderly or chronically ill people. Exposure to this toxin can produce severe diarrhea that results in marked fluid losses and frank shock.

Ricin

Ricin and aflatoxin are plant-derived toxins. Ricin is a poison that can be made from the waste left over from processing castor beans. It can be in the form of a powder, a mist, or a pellet, or it can be dissolved in water or weak acid. It is not affected much by extreme conditions, such as very hot or very cold temperatures.

It would take a deliberate act to make ricin and use it to poison people. Accidental exposure to ricin is highly unlikely. People can breathe in ricin mist or powder and be poisoned. Ricin also can get into water or food and be swallowed. Pellets of ricin or ricin dissolved in a liquid can be injected into people's bodies. Depending on the route of exposure (eg, injection or inhalation), 500 μg of ricin could be enough to kill an adult. A 500-μg dose of ricin would be about the size of the head of a pin. A greater amount likely would be needed to kill people if ricin were swallowed. Effects of ricin poisoning depend on whether ricin was inhaled, ingested, or injected. The major symptoms of ricin poisoning depend on the route of exposure and the dose received, although many organs may be affected in severe cases.

In 1978, Georgi Markov, a Bulgarian writer and journalist who was living in London, died after he was attacked by a man with an umbrella. The umbrella had been rigged to inject a poison ricin pellet under Markov's skin. Some reports have indicated that ricin may have been used in the Iran-Iraq war during the 1980s.

Initial symptoms of ricin poisoning by inhalation may occur within 8 hours of exposure. After ingestion of ricin, initial symptoms typically occur in less than 6 hours. Inhalation of ricin produces weakness, fever, cough, and pulmonary edema within 24 hours, with death from hypoxemia occurring in 36 to 72 hours. When ingested, ricin produces severe vomiting and diarrhea, resulting in cardiovascular collapse. Treatment is supportive; there is no antidote.

Treatment for children exposed to bioterrorism agents

Recommended medications can be used in response to category A agents despite the lack of FDA indications for some medications and relative contraindications for others. These recommendations include FDA-indicated medications, medications that do not have an FDA indication for children but literature and medical judgment support their usage, acceptable alternatives, and medications with valid reasons for use despite relative contraindications (Tables 2 and 3). As part of effective pediatric preparedness for bioterrorism events, one not only must have these agents for pediatric usage, but also must maintain them in forms that allow pediatric administration. This preparedness not only includes the availability of liquid preparations, but also staff and facilities for dosing to accommodate different-weight children and to reconstitute the liquid medications.

In addition to the medications described in the event of bioterrorism, one may have to consider immunotherapy and immunoprophylaxis. There are also unique pediatric considerations for these agents, including many that are not used or may not be FDA indicated for children (Box 3).

Surveillance

One of the key elements in terrorism preparedness is early detection of any possible terrorism event. The most likely scenario involves exposure in a community that may manifest with subtle symptoms and signs and unusual patient presentations in terms of numbers of diseases. Physicians must function constantly as part of a surveillance system to provide for early detection of any bioterrorism agent.

To enhance detection and treatment capabilities, health care providers should be familiar with the clinical manifestations, diagnostic techniques, isolation precautions, treatment, and prophylaxis for likely causative agents. They also must become familiar with referral procedures and when to report to the local health department. Health department reporting is based on local requirements, but should be considered for all unusual cases, including any cases suspicious for a terrorist agent or an unusual number of patients either absolute or for the season presenting with similar symptoms.

For some of these agents, delay in medical response could result in a potentially devastating number of casualties. Physicians must have an increased level of suspicion regarding the possible intentional use of biologic

Table 2
Recommended therapy and prophylaxis of anthrax in children

Form of anthrax	Category of treatment (therapy or prophylaxis)	Agent and dosage
Inhalational	Therapy[a] Patients who are clinically stable after 14 d can be switched to a single oral agent (ciprofloxacin or doxycycline) to complete a 60-day course[b] of therapy	Ciprofloxacin[c] 10–15 mg/kg IV q12h (max 400 mg/dose) *or* Doxycycline 2.2 mg/kg IV (max 100 mg) q12h *and* Clindamycin[d] 10–15 mg/kg IV q8h *and* Penicillin G[e] 400,000–600,000 U/kg/d IV divided q4h
Inhalational	Postexposure prophylaxis (60-day course[b])	Ciprofloxacin[f] 10–15 mg/kg PO (max 500 mg/dose) q12h *or* Doxycycline 2.2 mg/kg (max 100 mg) PO q12h
Cutaneous, endemic	Therapy[g]	Penicillin V 40–80 mg/kg/d PO divided q6h *or* Amoxicillin 40–80 mg/kg/d PO divided q8h *or* Ciprofloxacin 10–15 mg/kg PO (max 1 g/d) q12h *or* Doxycycline 2.2 mg/kg PO (max 100 mg) q12h
Cutaneous (In setting of terrorism)	Therapy[g]	Ciprofloxacin 10–15 mg/kg PO (max 1 g/d) q12h *or* Doxycycline 2.2 mg/kg PO (max 100 mg) q12h
Gastrointestinal	Therapy[a]	Same as for inhalational

Recommendations developed by the Columbia University Mailman School of Public Health National Center for Disaster Preparedness at the Pediatric Disaster and Terrorism National Consensus Conference.

[a] In a mass casualty setting in which resources are severely limited, oral therapy may need to be substituted for the preferred parenteral option. This may be most acceptable for ciprofloxacin because it is rapidly and well absorbed from the gastrointestinal tract with no substantial loss from first-pass effect.

[b] Children may be switched to oral amoxicillin (40–80 mg/kg/d divided q8h) to complete a 60-day course (assuming the organism is sensitive). We recommend that the first 14 days of therapy or postexposure prophylaxis, however, include ciprofloxacin or doxycycline or both regardless of age. A three-dose series of vaccine may permit shortening of the antibiotic course to 30 days.

[c] Levofloxacin or ofloxacin may be acceptable alternatives to ciprofloxacin.

[d] Rifampin or clarithromycin may be acceptable alternatives to clindamycin as drugs that target bacterial protein synthesis. If ciprofloxacin or another quinolone is used, doxycycline may be used as a second agent because it also targets protein synthesis.

[e] Ampicillin, imipenem, meropenem, or chloramphenicol may be acceptable alternatives to penicillin as drugs with good central nervous system penetration.

[f] According to most experts, ciprofloxacin is the preferred agent for oral prophylaxis.

[g] 10 days of therapy may be adequate for endemic cutaneous disease. A full 60-day course is recommended, however, in the setting of terrorism because of the possibility of concomitant inhalational exposure.

Adapted from Markenson D, Redlener I. Pediatric Disaster and Terrorism National Consensus Conference: executive summary. New York: National Center for Disaster Preparedness; 2003. p. 40.

Table 3
Recommended therapy and prophylaxis in children for additional select diseases associated with bioterrorism

Disease	Therapy or prophylaxis	Treatment, agent, and dosage[a]
Smallpox	Therapy	Supportive care
	Prophylaxis	Vaccination may be effective if given within the first several days after exposure
Plague	Therapy	Gentamicin 2.5 mg/kg IV q8h *or* Streptomycin 15 mg/kg IM q12h (max 2 g/d, although available only for compassionate usage and in limited supply is a preferred agent) *or* Doxycycline 2.2 mg/kg IV q12h (max 200 mg/d) *or* Ciprofloxacin 15 mg/kg IV q12h *or* Chloramphenicol[b] 25 m/kg q6h (max 4 g/d)
	Prophylaxis	Doxycycline 2.2 mg/kg PO q12h *or* Ciprofloxacin[c] 20 mg/kg PO q12h
Tularemia	Therapy	Same as for plague
Botulism	Therapy	Supportive care, antitoxin may halt progression of symptoms, but is unlikely to reverse them
Viral hemorrhagic fevers	Therapy	Supportive care, ribavirin may be beneficial in select cases[d]
Brucellosis	Therapy[e]	TMP/SMX 30 mg/kg PO q12h and rifampin 15 mg/kg q24h or gentamicin 7.5 mg/kg IM qd × 5

Recommendations developed by the Columbia University Mailman School of Public Health National Center for Disaster Preparedness at the Pediatric Disaster and Terrorism National Consensus Conference.

[a] In a mass casualty setting, parenteral therapy might not be possible. In such cases, oral therapy (with analogous agents) may need to be used.

[b] Concentration should be maintained between 5 and 20 μg/mL. Some experts have recommended that chloramphenicol be used to treat patients with plague meningitis because chloramphenicol penetrates the blood-brain barrier. Use in children <2 years old may be associated with adverse reactions but might be warranted for serious infections.

[c] Other fluoroquinolones (levofloxacin, ofloxacin) may be acceptable substitutes for ciprofloxacin; however, they are not approved for use in children.

[d] Ribavirin is recommended for arenavirus and bunyavirus and may be indicated for a viral hemorrhagic fever of an unknown etiology, although not approved by the Food and Drug Administration for these indications. For intravenous therapy, use a loading dose: 30 kg IV once (maximum dose 2 g), then 16 mg/kg IV every 6 hours for 4 days (maximum dose, 1 g) and then 8 mg/kg IV every 8 hours for 6 days (maximum dose, 500 mg). In a mass casualty setting, it may be necessary to use oral therapy. For oral therapy, use a loading dose of 30 mg/kg once, then 15 mg/kg/day in two divided doses for 10 days.

[e] For children <8 years old. For children >8 years old, adult regimens are recommended. Oral drugs should be given for 6 weeks. Gentamicin, if used, should be given for the first 5 days of a 6-week course of trimethoprim-sulfamethoxazole (TMP-SMX).

Adapted from Markenson D, Redlener I. Pediatric Disaster and Terrorism National Consensus Conference: executive summary. New York: National Center for Disaster Preparedness; 2003. p. 41.

Box 3. Immunotherapy and immunoprophylaxis

Anthrax

The currently licensed anthrax vaccine (Anthrax Vaccine Adsorbed, AVA; Bioport, Lansing, MI) is approved for persons 18–65 years old. This vaccine may have a limited role as an adjunct to postexposure chemoprophylaxis, although data are limited. In such an event, potential benefit would have to be weighed against unproven risk to children. There is limited potential for use of this vaccine in a civilian pre-exposure setting, but future studies of new-generation vaccines should include children.

Smallpox

The currently licensed smallpox vaccine (Dryvax; Wyeth, Philadelphia, PA) makes no mention in its package insert of an approved age range. In practice, until the early 1970s, this vaccine was administered to 1-year-olds. The Centers for Disease Control and Prevention (CDC) currently recommends against vaccination of children <1 year old. All contraindications to smallpox vaccination are relative. After bona fide exposure or known usage of weaponized smallpox, all exposed at-risk infants should be vaccinated. Future studies of new-generation vaccines must include children.

Botulism

A licensed trivalent (types A, B, E) antitoxin is available through the CDC. This antitoxin is to be used in children of any age known to have been exposed to botulinum toxin of the appropriate serotypes. An IND pentavalent (types A–E) Botulinum Immune Globulin (human) is available through the California Department of Health specifically for the treatment of infantile botulism. The study of this product must be continued and licensure pursued.

Plague

No licensed plague vaccine is currently in production. A previously licensed vaccine was approved only for persons 18–61 years old. There is little, if any, role for this or similar vaccines in a bioterrorist context.

Recommendations developed by the Columbia University Mailman School of Public Health National Center for Disaster Preparedness at the Pediatric Disaster and Terrorism National Consensus Conference.

Adapted from Markenson D, Redlener I. Pediatric Disaster and Terrorism National Consensus Conference: executive summary. New York: National Center for Disaster Preparedness; 2003.

Box 4. Important clues that may signal a biologic emergency

- A single suspected case of an uncommon disease
- Single or multiple cases of a suspected common disease or syndrome that does not respond to treatment as expected
- Clusters of a similar illness occurring in the same time frame in different locales
- Unusual clinical, geographical, seasonal, or temporal presentation of a disease or unusual transmission route
- Unexplained increase in incidence of an endemic disease
- Unusual illness that affects a large disparate population or is unusual for a population or age group
- Unusual pattern of illness or death among animals or humans
- Sudden increase in the following nonspecific illnesses: pneumonia; flulike illness; fever with atypical features; bleeding disorders; unexplained rashes and mucosal or skin irritation, particularly in adults; neuromuscular illness, such as muscle weakness and paralysis; or diarrhea

Adapted from Management of public health emergencies—a resource guide for physicians and other community responders [CD-ROM]. Chicago (IL): American Medical Association; 2005.

agents and an increased sensitivity to reporting those suspicions to public health authorities. Clinicians should report noticeable increases in unusual illnesses, symptom complexes, or disease patterns (even without definitive diagnosis) to public health authorities (Box 4).

Further readings

American Academy of Pediatrics. Children terrorism and disaster resource. Available at: http://www.aap.org/terrorism. Accessed June 30, 2005.

Centers for Disease Control and Prevention. Emergency preparedness and response. Available at: http://www.bt.cdc.gov. Accessed June 30, 2005.

Chemical-biological terrorism and its impact on children. Pediatrics 2002;105:662–70.

Lillibridge SR, Bell AJ, Roman RS. Centers for Disease Control and Prevention bioterrorism preparedness and response. Am J Infect Control 1999;27:463–4.

Markenson D, Redlener I. Pediatric Disaster and Terrorism National Consensus Conference: executive summary. New York: National Center for Disaster Preparedness; 2003.

Redlener I, Markenson D. Disaster and terrorism preparedness: what pediatricians need to know. Adv Pediatr 2003;50:1–37.

ELSEVIER
SAUNDERS

Infect Dis Clin N Am 19 (2005) 747–757

INFECTIOUS
DISEASE CLINICS
OF NORTH AMERICA

Implications of Methicillin-Resistant *Staphylococcus aureus* as a Community-Acquired Pathogen in Pediatric Patients

Sheldon L. Kaplan, MD[a,b,*]

[a]*Department of Pediatrics, Baylor College of Medicine, Houston, TX 77030, USA*
[b]*Infectious Disease Service, Texas Children's Hospital, Feigin Center MC 3-2371, Suite 1150, 1102 Bates, Houston, TX 77030, USA*

Methicillin-resistant *Staphylococcus aureus* (MRSA) is now an established community pathogen in many areas of the United States and the world [1–5]. Community-acquired MRSA (CA-MRSA) infections have changed several aspects of staphylococcal infections in children, including the epidemiology, clinical manifestations, laboratory diagnosis, treatment, and prevention.

Epidemiology

The incidence of *S aureus* infections in children is unknown because this determination depends on specific culture data, and until more recently, most skin and soft tissue infections were treated empirically without cultures being obtained. Nevertheless, in a Centers for Disease Control and Prevention study examining CA-MRSA infections in 2001–2002, the incidence for white children and black children younger than 2 years old was approximately 16/100,000 and 70/100,000 in Atlanta and 18/100,000 and 40/100,000 in Baltimore [6]. The incidence for white children and black children 2 to 18 years old was approximately 9/100,000 and 24/100,000 in Atlanta and 12/100,000 and 15/100,000 in Baltimore. Other investigators also have noted the differences in frequency of CA-MRSA infections among

* Infectious Disease Service, Texas Children's Hospital, Feigin Center MC 3-2371, Suite 1150, 1102 Bates, Houston, TX 77030, USA.
E-mail address: skaplan@bcm.tmc.edu

0891-5520/05/$ - see front matter
doi:10.1016/j.idc.2005.05.011 *id.theclinics.com*

different racial groups. In other regions, CA-MRSA infections are particularly common among Native Americans [2].

In several areas, the number of CA-MRSA infections is increasing in children, although how much is a real increase compared with physicians being more aggressive about obtaining cultures is unclear. At Texas Children's Hospital, the percentage of community-acquired *S aureus* isolates that are MRSA and the overall number of community-acquired *S aureus* isolates have increased significantly in the 3 years from August 1, 2001, to July 31, 2004 [7]. The percentage of community-acquired *S aureus* isolates resistant to methicillin increased from 72% to 76%, and the total number of isolates virtually doubled over 3 years (771 to 1562). Determining what factors are related to this increase in *S aureus* infections is under investigation, but may relate in part to specific virulence characteristics of the more common CA-MRSA clones in circulation. The clone designated USA300 by the Centers for Disease Control and Prevention is particularly capable of spreading rapidly when in the community [8].

CA-MRSA infections also seem to be more common among family members than has been seen in the past with community-acquired methicillin-susceptible *S aureus* (CA-MSSA) isolates. Spread among daycare attendees and athletes has been documented [9,10]. *S aureus* isolates with the characteristics associated with CA-MRSA isolates (SCC*mec* IV, presence of *pvl* genes, limited antimicrobial resistance) have been isolated from patients with nosocomial infections, including neonates in the neonatal intensive care unit [11,12].

Clinical manifestations

Skin and soft tissue infections constitute greater than 90% of the infections caused by CA-MRSA in children [1,2,6,7]. Cellulitis, abscesses, and folliculitis are the predominant skin infections. Head and neck CA-MRSA infections, such as cervical lymphadenitis, otitis externa, otitis media with otorrhea, and acute mastoiditis, also are being encountered with increasing frequency [13]. Recurrent skin infections are seen frequently in children with CA-MRSA infections. Most CA-MRSA isolates carry the genes encoding the cytotoxin Panton-Valentine leukocidin (PVL), which has been implicated as a factor in the possible enhanced ability of CA-MRSA isolates to cause skin infections [13–15]. PVL also may contribute to the ability of CA-MRSA isolates to cause more complicated infections at other sites.

Among the invasive infections caused by CA-MRSA isolates, musculoskeletal infections are the most common. At Texas Children's Hospital, acute hematogenous osteomyelitis now is caused most commonly by CA-MRSA isolates. Over the 3-year study previously mentioned, there were 54 and 28 children with CA-MRSA and CA-MSSA osteomyelitis [7]. The clinical manifestations of osteomyelitis caused by CA-MRSA versus

CA-MSSA isolates are different in that multiple sites of infection are more common in patients with CA-MRSA infection at Texas Children's Hospital. In the author's series, children with CA-MRSA osteomyelitis had a longer duration of fever and hospital stay than children with osteomyelitis caused by CA-MSSA isolates [16].

The presence of the *pvl* genes in community-acquired *S aureus* isolates was associated with laboratory and clinical differences among the author's patients with acute osteomyelitis. Children with *pvl*-positive isolates had greater measures of inflammation at admission and during hospitalization (white blood cell count, erythrocyte sedimentation rate, C-reactive protein), greater frequency of positive blood cultures, and greater frequency of subperiosteal or intraosseous abscesses than children whose isolates did not carry the *pvl* genes [17]. More complications of osteomyelitis, such as the development of chronic osteomyelitis or an associated deep venous thrombosis, were seen in the children with *pvl*-positive isolates [16]. Venous thrombophlebitis leading to septic pulmonary emboli and other sites of dissemination occurs more commonly with the CA-MRSA USA300 clone for reasons that are not yet determined. In these circumstances, anticoagulation may be warranted.

CA-MRSA isolates are isolated less commonly from children with septic arthritis than from children with acute osteomyelitis. Over the aforementioned 3-year study, CA-MRSA and CA-MSSA isolates were recovered from 9 and 10 children with septic arthritis. The clinical manifestations were no different for these two groups [7].

Myositis and pyomyositis are being recognized with increasing frequency in children with CA-MRSA infections, and as with osteomyelitis, multiple sites of muscle involvement are not unusual [17]. A concomitant osteomyelitis also is common [16]. In studies at Texas Children's Hospital, myositis or pyomyositis was seen in association with osteomyelitis in 28 of 45 children with *pvl*-positive isolates compared with 6 of 19 children with *pvl*-negative isolates ($P = .05$) [17]. These children typically complain of pain in the region with tenderness to palpation of the involved muscles. In large muscles of the extremities, swelling and warmth may be appreciated. Of imaging techniques, MRI generally shows the muscle involvement most readily (Fig. 1), and its increased use may explain in part the increasing recognition of this infection [18]. Because multiple sites of myositis/pyomyositis or osteomyelitis can occur, physicians must examine the patient carefully daily to detect areas of infection that may not have been appreciated even the previous day. Repeat imaging, weekly in some cases, may be necessary to show these areas of inflammation and abscess formation as they develop.

Necrotizing fasciitis caused by CA-MRSA has been described in adults, many of whom have chronic underlying illnesses [19]. It is likely that this manifestation of CA-MRSA infection also will be described in children.

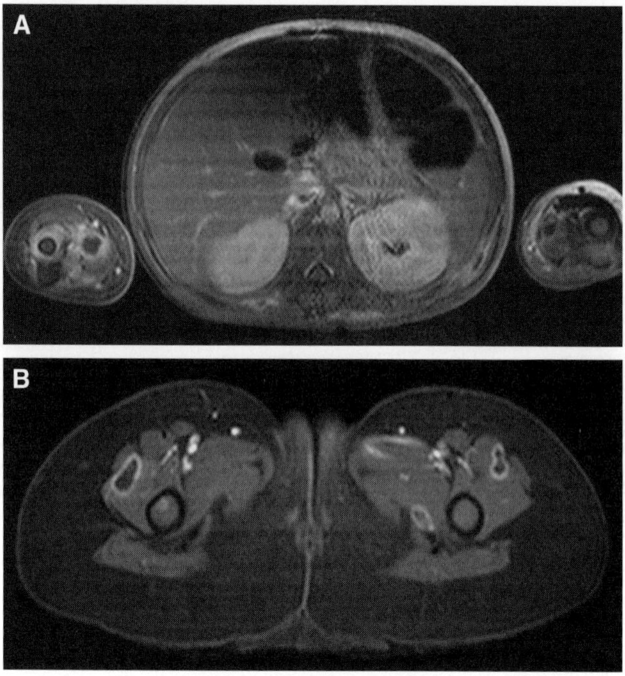

Fig. 1. (*A* and *B*) MRI of a child with multiple sites of pyomyositis caused by CA-MRSA.

Complicated pneumonias with empyema also have been encountered more frequently in children since CA-MRSA isolates have become so common. At Texas Children's Hospital, CA-MRSA is now the most common cause of pleural empyema in children [20]. Clinical findings for pneumonia with empyema are similar for CA-MRSA infections compared with other organisms, such as *Streptococcus pneumoniae*. The length of stay for children with CA-MRSA empyema was longer (mean 18.8 days), however, than seen in children with CA-MSSA empyema (mean 14 days). Children with primary CA-MRSA pneumonia are younger than children with CA-MRSA pulmonary manifestations associated with infections at other sites, typically bones or joints. Among children with invasive infections, community-acquired *S aureus* isolates carrying the genes encoding PVL are more likely to be associated with abnormal chest imaging than isolates negative for the *pvl* genes [21]. CA-MRSA isolates have been associated with a necrotizing pneumonia, especially in children coinfected with a respiratory virus [22]. The mortality rates for necrotizing pneumonia are quite high.

As CA-MRSA infections continue to increase, the number of children with severe invasive CA-MRSA infections also has increased in many areas [23,24]. At Texas Children's Hospital, from September 2002 through January 2004, about 10% (16 of 150) of the children with invasive community-acquired *S aureus* infections were admitted to the intensive care unit [25]. Fourteen of the 16 patients were older than age 10 years, with an average age of 12.9 years and mean weight of 63 kg. Focusing on the 14 older children, most had skeletal infections, bacteremia, and pulmonary involvement; 11 required mechanical ventilation. Four had vascular thromboses. The mean duration of bacteremia was 4 days (range 1–11 days), and the mean duration of fever was 13 days. Three of these 14 patients died. One of the two younger patients also died.

Despite the impressive increase in CA-MRSA infections overall and the invasive infections in particular, the author has not noted a remarkable increase in the number of children with infective endocarditis owing to this organism. Transthoracic echocardiograms are performed in virtually all patients with persistent bacteremia (>4 days), and in only a few children have vegetations been identified [25].

CA-MRSA isolates have been associated with a purpura fulminans presentation in adults and children similar to severe meningococcemia [26]. Rapid onset of purpura with the need for amputation of extremities with high mortality can occur [27]. The relationship of this clinical presentation to specific superantigens, such as TSST-1, SEB, or SEC, or the CA-MRSA clone (USA400 versus USA300) is unclear. Large spinal epidural abscesses spanning from the cervical to the lumbar regions caused by CA-MRSA isolates have been noted in several children at Texas Children's Hospital.

Laboratory studies

Microbiology laboratories have to be capable of rapidly identifying and providing antimicrobial susceptibility data for antibiotics appropriate for pediatric use. Using newer molecular techniques, the presence of the *mec*A gene now can be detected rapidly in isolates and possibly in patient specimens directly in the future [28]. Up-to-date information regarding the current antimicrobial susceptibility patterns of community-acquired *S aureus* isolates in a community is crucial to being able to treat patients with suspected staphylococcal infections most optimally. It is quite difficult, however, for laboratories to separate out community-acquired from health care–associated *S aureus* infections. Physicians are encouraged to obtain purulent specimens for culture for the benefit of the patient and for determining the proportion of MRSA among community-acquired *S aureus* isolates or at least to know the proportion in a specific office or clinic.

Vancomycin, trimethoprim-sulfamethoxazole (TMP-SMX), clindamycin, doxycycline, and linezolid should be included in the routine panel of agents tested. Detecting inducible macrolide-lincosamide-streptogramin B is recommended when clindamycin is an important option for treatment because treatment failures with clindamycin have been documented in patients treated for an invasive infection caused by *S aureus* isolates with inducible macrolide-lincosamide-streptogramin B resistance [29].

Clindamycin resistance among CA-MRSA isolates varies from 4% to 6% to 20% or greater in some regions.

Treatment

Skin and soft tissue infections

When CA-MRSA is an initial consideration as the cause of an infection or is isolated, β-lactam antibiotics, such as dicloxacillin or cephalexin for outpatients or nafcillin, oxacillin, or cefazolin for inpatients, are no longer appropriate for empirical treatment or for completing treatment. The optimal management of skin and soft tissue infections is unclear. Although incision and drainage of abscesses alone without antimicrobial therapy may be effective in many patients, particularly for abscesses less than 5 cm in diameter, antimicrobial therapy usually is still provided [30].

Empirical antistaphylococcal β-lactam antibiotic treatment for skin and soft tissue infections is not recommended in areas where CA-MRSA isolates are known to account for 10% to 15% or more of community isolates. In this setting, TMP-SMX or clindamycin can be employed [31]. Whether adding rifampin to TMP-SMX is beneficial in unknown. Clinical studies of TMP-SMX treatment of CA-MRSA infections are limited, although early clinical studies showed that TMP-SMX was effective in treating MSSA infections [32–34]. TMP-SMX is not active against group A streptococcus, another common cause of skin and soft tissue infections. TMP-SMX may result in hypersensitivity reactions or bone marrow suppression. There are no data on TMP-SMX treatment of invasive CA-MRSA infections in children. Doxycycline or minocycline has been efficacious in treating adults with skin and soft tissue infections secondary to MRSA and is a consideration for children older than age 8 years [35].

Invasive infections

Vancomycin is recommended for inclusion in initial empirical antibiotic regimens for seriously ill patients with infections that may be due to CA-MRSA. Gentamicin with or without rifampin frequently is added to vancomycin for suspected life-threatening MRSA infections. Nafcillin/oxacillin is more rapidly bactericidal than vancomycin for MSSA isolates, and clinical data in adults suggest that nafcillin/oxacillin is superior to vancomycin for the treatment of bacteremic pneumonia secondary to MSSA [36]. Nafcillin/oxacillin also is recommended in addition to vancomycin in the initial empirical regimen to cover for MSSA isolates optimally.

CA-MRSA isolates generally are susceptible to clindamycin and TMP-SMX, but regional differences occur. Clindamycin is efficacious in treating serious infections caused by clindamycin-susceptible CA-MRSA isolates, including osteomyelitis, septic arthritis, and pleural empyema [16,20,31,37,38]. Clindamycin is administered intravenously at a dose of 30 to

40 mg/kg/day in three divided doses. Clindamycin is well absorbed by the oral route, so treatment can be completed with oral clindamycin at the same dose. The most concerning adverse effect of clindamycin is *Clostridium difficile* enteritis, which is a relatively rare complication. Perhaps the most common effect is loose stools or diarrhea. Clindamycin also may be associated with a rash; the oral suspension of clindamycin is not very palatable.

In some regions of the United States, a high proportion of CA-MRSA strains are clindamycin resistant. If the proportion of CA-MRSA isolates resistant to clindamycin exceeds 10% to 15%, clindamycin should not be used for empirical treatment of suspected staphylococcal infections.

Linezolid is an oxazolidinone antibiotic that is equivalent to vancomycin for the treatment of serious MRSA infections, including bacteremia and pneumonia in children [39]. Linezolid has not been studied in the treatment of osteomyelitis, but case reports or series and a compassionate use summary suggest linezolid is effective in treating osteomyelitis caused by MRSA [40,41]. The main side effect of linezolid is diarrhea; thrombocytopenia, optic neuritis, and neuropathy may occur with prolonged administration. Linezolid is well absorbed after oral administration, and therapy can be completed with an oral formulation at the same dose as given intravenously. Daptomycin is approved for the treatment of serious staphylococcal infections in adults, but may not be efficacious in treating pulmonary infection [42]. The dosage and safety profile of daptomycin are unknown in children. The American Academy of Pediatrics has outlined an approach to managing suspected CA-MRSA skin and soft tissue infections and more invasive infections (Fig. 2) [43].

Aggressive drainage of abscesses or other purulent collections is crucial to the successful management of these patients. Surgical incision and drainage of large abscesses in soft tissue or intraosseous/subperiosteal collections is ideal. Drainage by an interventional radiologist may suffice or may be the only way to approach safely some abscesses in deep locations, especially in critically ill children. In these situations, infectious disease and critical care medicine physicians have to remain in close communication with general surgery or orthopedic surgery colleagues to facilitate the optimal timing for these drainage procedures. MRI is invaluable for locating and showing these collections so that the surgeons can plan the approach to drainage most optimally. The value of adjunctive therapies, such as intravenous immunoglobulin preparations enriched for antibodies against specific toxins or surface proteins of *S aureus*, is under investigation [44].

Prevention

Prompt attention to cuts, abrasions, or other injuries to the skin, such as keeping the area clean and dry and applying a topical antibiotic at the first sign of inflammation, may help prevent superficial infections. Recurrent

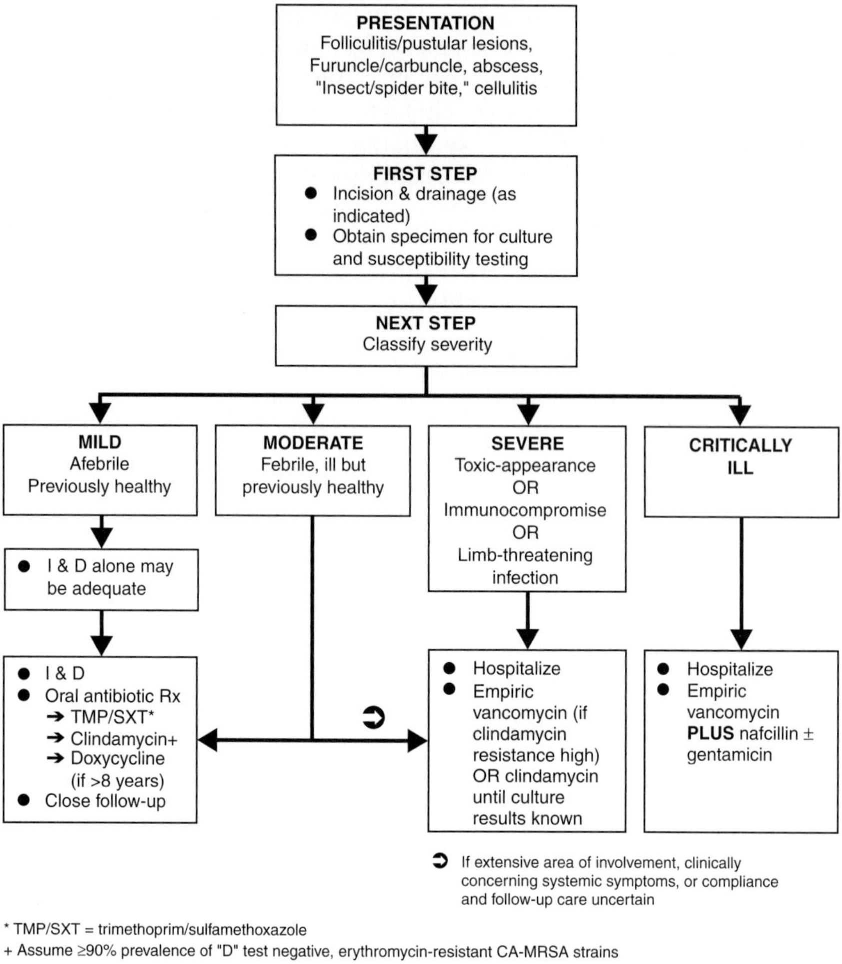

Fig. 2. Algorithm for managing children with suspected CA-MRSA infections suggested by the American Academy of Pediatrics. Initial outpatient management of suspected CA-MRSA skin and soft tissue infections is schematically illustrated and assumes CA-MRSA strains are prevalent in a community. (*Data from* Baker CJ, Frenck RW Jr. Change in management of skin/soft tissue infections needed. AAP News 2004;25:10.)

CA-MRSA infections in a child and CA-MRSA infections among multiple family members are quite common. Keeping fingernails clean and cut short and changing towels, washcloths, underwear, and sleepwear daily are reasonable measures to recommend. Applying mupirocin to the anterior nares may be useful to diminish nasal colonization by CA-MRSA, although a Cochrane review did not find topical antibiotics to be useful for eradicating nasal MRSA [45]. Resistance to mupirocin is increasing worldwide [46]. Finally, taking a bath twice a week for 15 minutes in water to which regular-strength Clorox bleach (1 teaspoon per 1 gallon of water) has been added seems to be helpful in preventing recurrent infections in the author's experience.

References

[1] Herold BC, Immergluck LC, Maranan MC, et al. Community-acquired methicillin-resistant *Staphylococcus aureus* in children with no identified predisposing risk. JAMA 1998;279: 593–8.

[2] Naimi TS, LeDell KH, Boxrud DJ, et al. Epidemiology and clonality of community-acquired methicillin-resistant *Staphylococcus aureus* in Minnesota, 1996–1998. Clin Infect Dis 2001;33:990–6.

[3] Purcell K, Fergie JE. Exponential increase in community-acquired methicillin-resistant *Staphylococcus aureus* infections in South Texas children. Pediatr Infect Dis J 2002;21:988–9.

[4] Buckingham SC, McDougal LK, Cathey LD, et al. Emergence of community-associated methicillin-resistant *Staphylococcus aureus* at a Memphis, Tennessee Children's Hospital. Pediatr Infect Dis J 2004;23:619–24.

[5] Sattler CA, Mason EO Jr, Kaplan SL. Prospective comparison of risk factors and demographic and clinical characteristics of community-acquired, methicillin-resistant versus methicillin-susceptible *Staphylococcus aureus* infection in children. Pediatr Infect Dis J 2002; 21:910–7.

[6] Fridkin SK, Hageman JC, Morrison M, et al. Methicillin-resistant *Staphylococcus aureus* disease in three communities. N Engl J Med 2005;352:1436–44.

[7] Kaplan SL, Hulten KG, Gonzalez BE, et al. Three years' surveillance of community-acquired *Staphylococcus aureus* infections in children. Clin Infect Dis 2005;40:1785–91.

[8] McDougal LK, Steward CD, Killgore GE, Chaitram JM, McAllister SK, Tenover FC. Pulsed-field gel electrophoresis typing of oxacillin-resistant *Staphylococcus aureus* isolates from the United States: establishing a national database. J Clin Microbiol 2003;41:5113–20.

[9] Centers for Disease Control. Methicillin-resistant *Staphylococcus aureus* infections among competitive sports participants—Colorado, Indiana, Pennsylvania, and Los Angeles County, 2000–2003. MMWR Morb Mortal Wkly Rep 2000;52:793–5.

[10] Adcock PM, Pastor P, Medley F, Patterson JE, Murphy TV. Methicillin-resistance *Staphylococcus aureus* in two child care centers. J Infect Dis 1998;178:577–80.

[11] Carleton HA, Diep BA, Charlebois ED, et al. Community-adapted methicillin-resistant *Staphylococcus aureus* (MRSA): population dynamics of an expanding community reservoir of MRSA. J Infect Dis 2004;190:1730–8.

[12] Healy CM, Hulten KG, Palazzi DL, Campbell JR, Baker CJ. Emergence of new strains of methicillin-resistant *Staphylococcus aureus* in a neonatal intensive care unit. Clin Infect Dis 2004;39:1460–6.

[13] Santos FAB, Mankarious LA, Eavey RD. Methicillin-resistant *Staphylococcus aureus*: pediatric otitis. Arch Otolaryngol Head Neck Surg 2000;126:1383–5.

[14] Vandenesch F, Naimi T, Enright MC, et al. Community-acquired methicillin-resistant *Staphylococcus aureus* carrying Panton-Valentine leukocidin genes: worldwide emergence. Emerg Infect Dis 2003;9:978–84.

[15] Mishaan AMA, Mason EO Jr, Martinez-Aguilar G, et al. Emergence of a predominant clone of community *Staphylococcus aureus* among children in Houston, Texas. Pediatr Infect Dis J 2005;24:201–6.

[16] Martinez-Aguilar G, Avalos-Mishaan A, Hulten K, et al. Community-acquired, methicillin-resistant and methicillin-susceptible *Staphylococcus aureus* musculoskeletal infections in children. Pediatr Infect Dis J 2004;23:701–6.

[17] Bocchini CE, Hulten KG, Mason EO Jr, et al. Panton-Valentine leukocidin genes are associated with enhanced inflammatory response and local disease in acute hematogenous *Staphylococcus aureus* osteomyelitis in children. Pediatrics, in press.

[18] Trusen A, Beissert M, Schultz G, et al. Ultrasound and MRI features of pyomyositis in children. Eur Radiol 2003;13:1050–5.
[19] Miller LG, Perdreau-Remington F, Rieg G, et al. Necrotizing fasciitis caused by community-associated methicillin-resistant *Staphylococcus aureus* in Los Angeles. N Engl J Med 2005; 352:1445–53.
[20] Schultz KD, Fan LF, Pinsky J, et al. The changing face of pleural empyemas in children: epidemiology and management. Pediatrics 2004;113:1735–40.
[21] Gonzalez BE, Hulten KG, Dishop MK, et al. Pulmonary manifestations in children with invasive community-acquired *Staphylococcus aureus* infections. Clin Infect Dis, in press.
[22] Gillet Y, Issartel B, Vanhems P, et al. Association between *Staphylococcus aureus* strains carrying gene for Panton-Valentine leukocidin and highly lethal necrotizing pneumonia in young immunocompetent patients. Lancet 2002;359:753–9.
[23] Centers for Disease Control and Prevention. Four pediatric deaths from community-acquired methicillin-resistant *Staphylococcus aureus*—Minnesota and North Dakota, 1997–1999. JAMA 1999;282:1123–5.
[24] Mongkolrattanothai K, Boyle S, Kahana MD, Daum RS. Severe *Staphylococcus aureus* infections caused by clonally related community-acquired methicillin-susceptible and methicillin-resistant isolates. Clin Infect Dis 2003;37:1050–8.
[25] Gonzalez BE, Martinez-Aguilar G, Hulten KG, et al. Severe staphylococcal sepsis in adolescents in the era of community-acquired methicillin-resistant *Staphylococcus aureus*. Pediatrics 2005;115:642–8.
[26] Valente AM, Jain R, Scheurer M, et al. Frequency of infective endocarditis among infants and children with *Staphylococcus aureus* bacteremia. Pediatrics 2005;115:e15–9.
[27] Kravitz GR, Dries DJ, Peterson ML, Schlievert PM. Purpura fulminans due to *Staphylococcus aureus*. Clin Infect Dis 2005;40:941–7.
[28] Warren DK, Liao RS, Merz LR, Eveland M, Dunne WM Jr. Detection of methicillin-resistant *Staphylococcus aureus* directly from nasal swab specimens by a real-time PCR assay. J Clin Microbiol 2004;42:5578–81.
[29] Lewis JS II, Jorgensen JH. Inducible clindamycin resistance in staphylococci: should clinicians and microbiologists be concerned? Clin Infect Dis 2005;40:280–5.
[30] Lee MC, Riso AM, Aten MF, et al. Management and outcome of children with skin and soft tissue abscesses caused by community-acquired methicillin-resistant *Staphylococcus aureus*. Pediatr Infect Dis J 2004;23:123–7.
[31] Marcinak JF, Frank AL. Treatment of community-acquired methicillin-resistant *Staphylococcus aureus* in children. Curr Opin Infect Dis 2003;16:265–9.
[32] Adra M, Lawrence KR. Trimethoprim/sulfamethoxazole for treatment of severe *Staphylococcus aureus* infections. Ann Pharmacother 2004;38:338–41.
[33] Iyer S, Jones DH. Community-acquired methicillin-resistant *Staphylococcus aureus* skin infections: a retrospective analysis of clinical presentation and treatment of a local outbreak. J Am Acad Dermatol 2004;50:854–8.
[34] Ardati KO, Thirumoorthi MC, Dajani AS. Intravenous trimethoprim-sulfamethoxazole in the treatment of serious infections in children. J Pediatr 1979;95:801–6.
[35] Yuk JH, Dignani MC, Harris RL, Bradshaw MW, Williams TW Jr. Minocycline as an alternative antistaphylococcal agent. Rev Infect Dis 1991;13:1023–4.
[36] Gonzalez C, Rubio M, Romero-Vivas J, et al. Bacteremic pneumonia due to *Staphylococcus aureus*: a comparison of disease caused by methicillin-resistant and methicillin-susceptible organisms. Clin Infect Dis 1999;29:1171–7.
[37] Frank AL, Marcinak JF, Mangat PD, et al. Clindamycin treatment of methicillin-resistant *Staphylococcus aureus* infections in children. Pediatr Infect Dis J 2002;21:530–4.
[38] Martinez-Aguilar G, Hammerman WA, Mason EO Jr, Kaplan SL. Clindamycin treatment of invasive infections caused by community-acquired, methicillin- resistant and methicillin-susceptible *Staphylococcus aureus* in children. Pediatr Infect Dis J 2003;22: 593–8.

[39] Kaplan SL, Deville JG, Yogev R, et al. Linezolid versus vancomycin for treatment of resistant gram-positive infections in children. Pediatr Infect Dis J 2003;22:677–86.

[40] Rayner CR, Baddour LM, Birmingham MC, et al. Linezolid in the treatment of osteomyelitis: results of compassionate use experience. Infection 2004;32:8–14.

[41] Rao N, Ziran BH, Hall RA, Santa ER. Successful treatment of chronic bone and joint infections with oral linezolid. Clin Orthop 2004;427:67–71.

[42] Arbeit RD, Maki D, Tally FP, et al. The safety and efficacy of daptomycin for the treatment of complicated skin and skin-structure infections. Clin Infect Dis 2004;38:1673–81.

[43] Baker CJ, Frenck RW Jr. Change in management of skin/soft tissue infections needed. AAP News 2004;25:105.

[44] Gauduchon V, Cozon G, Vandenesch F, et al. Neutralization of *Staphylococcus aureus* Panton Valentine leukocidin by intravenous immunoglobulin in vitro. J Infect Dis 2004;189: 346–53.

[45] Chen SF. *Staphylococcus aureus* decolonization. Pediatr Infect Dis J 2005;24:70–80.

[46] Deshpande LM, Fix AM, Pfaller MA, et al. Emerging elevated mupirocin resistance rates among staphylococcal isoaltes in the SENTRY antimicrobial surveillance program (2000): correlations of results from disk diffusion, Etest and reference dilution methods. Diagn Microbiol Infect Dis 2002;42:283–90.

ELSEVIER
SAUNDERS

INFECTIOUS DISEASE CLINICS OF NORTH AMERICA

Infect Dis Clin N Am 19 (2005) 759–764

Index

Note: Page numbers of article titles are in **boldface** type.

doi:10.1016/S0891-5520(05)00086-3

Changing Your Address?

Make sure your subscription changes too! When you notify us of your new address, you can help make our job easier by including an exact copy of your Clinics label number with your old address (see illustration below.) This number identifies you to our computer system and will speed the processing of your address change. Please be sure this label number accompanies your old address and your corrected address—you can send an old Clinics label with your number on it or just copy it exactly and send it to the address listed below.

We appreciate your help in our attempt to give you continuous coverage. Thank you.

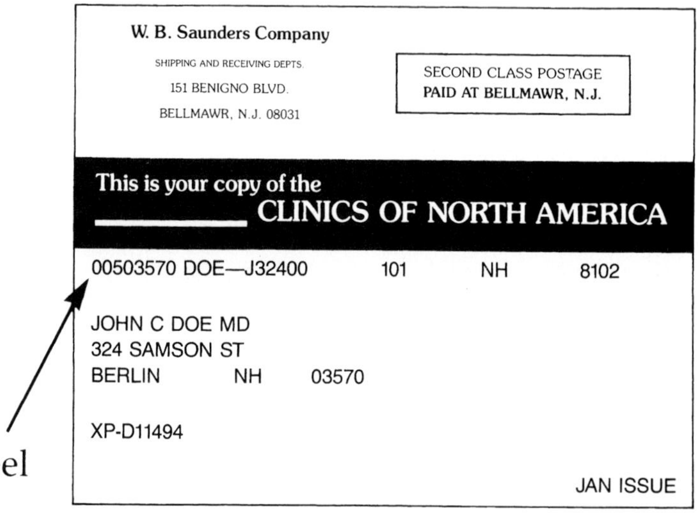
W. B. Saunders Company
SHIPPING AND RECEIVING DEPTS.
151 BENIGNO BLVD.
BELLMAWR, N.J. 08031

SECOND CLASS POSTAGE
PAID AT BELLMAWR, N.J.

This is your copy of the
________ CLINICS OF NORTH AMERICA

00503570 DOE—J32400 101 NH 8102

JOHN C DOE MD
324 SAMSON ST
BERLIN NH 03570

XP-D11494

JAN ISSUE

Your Clinics Label Number

Copy it exactly or send your label along with your address to:
W.B. Saunders Company, Customer Service
Orlando, FL 32887-4800
Call Toll Free 1-800-654-2452

Please allow four to six weeks for delivery of new subscriptions and for processing address changes.